WHAT READERS
THIS HAND~~BOOK~~...

'Without reservation, I highly recommend this book, and the writer. I will be using it in the Aspire Leisure Centre gym and recommending it to my colleagues. I am very proud of Caroline and her journey to where she is today. She is an inspiration to anyone with scoliosis. This book will help others with general spinal problems too.'

Liz Bord, Senior Exercise Specialist, Aspire Leisure Centre, Royal National Orthopaedic Hospital, Stanmore UK

'a great read. ...Section 3 will really help and it gives great practical advice.

Dean Tearle, Centre Manager, Aspire Leisure Centre
www.aspireleisurecentre.org.uk

'This book will be really helpful for a lot of people'

Stewart Tucker FRCS, Consultant spinal surgeon, Great Ormond Street Hospital and Royal National Orthopaedic Hospital, UK

'Thank you for sharing. This book is:
- *Easy and enjoyable to read*
- *Great idea and well delivered*
- *Pages 35 to 118 will be the most useful for gym instructors/physios/ personal trainers*
- *Lots of variety of exercises and good amount of detail given (with pictures) explaining how to do the exercises and why.'*

Gemma Bruce, Extended Scope Practitioner, Spinal Deformities, Royal National Orthopaedic Hospital

THE SCOLIOSIS HANDBOOK

OF SAFE AND EFFECTIVE EXERCISES PRE AND POST SURGERY

To Alex and Zoe

THE SCOLIOSIS HANDBOOK

OF SAFE AND EFFECTIVE EXERCISES PRE AND POST SURGERY

CAROLINE FREEDMAN

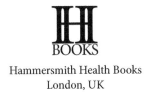

Hammersmith Health Books
London, UK

First published in 2020 by Hammersmith Health Books – an imprint of
Hammersmith Books Limited
4/4A Bloomsbury Square, London WC1A 2RP, UK
www.hammersmithbooks.co.uk

Reprinted 2021

Disclaimer: The information provided in this book is for educational purposes only.
It is the result of the study and experience of the author. This book is not meant
to be used, nor should it be used, to diagnose or treat any medical condition. For
diagnosis or treatment of any medical problem, always consult your own physician.
The publisher and author are not responsible for any specific health or allergy
needs that may require medical supervision and are not liable for any damages or
negative consequences from any treatment, action, application or preparation, to
any person reading or following the information in this book. Any references are
provided for informational purposes only and do not constitute endorsement of
any websites or other sources. Readers should be aware that the websites included
in this book may change.

Print ISBN: 978-1-78161-166-1
Ebook ISBN: 978-1-78161-167-8

Designed and typeset by: Hannah Robinson, Dunelm Digital and Julie Bennett,
Bespoke Publishing Ltd.
Commissioning Editor: Georgina Bentliff
Cover design by: Hannah Robinson, Dunelm Digital
Cover photo by: Sam Pearce
Portrait photos provided: of Nicki Waterman by Stewart Williams, of the author by
Sam Pearce of Square Image. Liz Bord, John Rutherford and Zeinab Choudhury
provided their portraits.
Production: Helen Whitehorn, Path Projects Ltd
Printed and bound by: TJ Books Limited

Contents

Acknowledgements

I would like to thank the following people for their invaluable support over the years of my scoliosis journey:

My sweet Mum who nursed me through my surgeries. Calm, patient, loving and always able to understand absolutely how I was feeling at any moment. My Dad who was there supporting both of us and always strong (except for the donating blood bit).

Alex and Zoe, the reason I had the surgery in the first place was to make sure I could have you both. You are my complete world. Alex, I loved you making breakfast for me every morning when I first came home after the last surgery and making sure I wasn't left alone. Zoe, always giving me time, whatever you were doing. Small things like going shopping and coming home with gadgets so I didn't slip over in the shower show your kindness and meant so much. I love you both.

Jeremy Jel, the best brother who wrote off my car while I was having surgery – love you!

Julia, my rock. You found my scoliosis and you have always been there for everything, like a sister and more. My friends Sarah and Suzanne, with me through everything, and all my other friends and family who were kind and gave me their time.

Tony, with me for the first two surgeries, I am forever grateful for your love and care at that time. Your bravery is incredible.

Stephen, my husband, for your support, love and care through the last surgery. For encouraging me and giving me the space to write this guide. I love you, Daniella and Josh.

My clients who still came to me when I could only point out a Personal Training class after surgery.

My two surgeons, Mr Michael Edgar and Mr Stewart Tucker. My many physios, including John Rutherford who continues to take away any pain and has contributed an introduction and a number of exercises to this book. Staff at The London Clinic and The Wellington Hospital. Mr Hilali Noordeen, my daughter Zoe's consultant. Mr Jan Lehovsky. Mr Peter Mason FRCS FRCOG, consultant obstetrician and gynaecologist.

Liz Bord at Aspire Leisure Centre (within the grounds of the RNOH) – without your suggestion, this guide would have just been an A4 piece of paper. Dean Tearle: Aspire Leisure Centre - thank you for your support.

Nicki Waterman (1964–2016)
Photography: Sam Pearce, Square Image
Illustrator: Hannah Robinson, Dunelm Digital (see page 141)
Proofreader: Ruth Burns Warrens – really appreciate your helpful editing advice.
Editing advice: Caroline at Caroline Ratner Communications
Sharon Portner at the Film Company – thank you for proofing and testing the exercises.
Design and typesetting: Julie Bennett – thank you so much for your invaluable expertise designing and creating my handbook.
Publisher: Hammersmith Books – Georgina Bentliff – I am so grateful to you for believing in my book from the start and for all your worthy, much appreciated professional guidance and advice in polishing this manuscript. A huge thank you.

Foreword by Liz Bord

Senior Cardiac Rehabilitation
Exercise Specialist,
Aspire Leisure Centre,
Royal National Orthopaedic Hospital,
Stanmore, UK

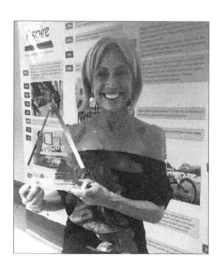 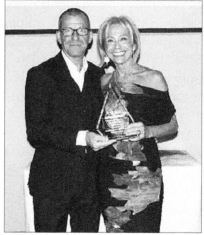

Liz Bord receiving The Spirit of Aspire award in 2016

My name is Elizabeth Bord and I have worked for the charity Aspire for 26 years. Aspire works with people who have been paralysed by spinal cord injury, supporting them from injury to independence.

The charity specialises in supporting people with spinal injuries through integration, rehabilitation, education, housing etc. I work in the gym and during this time have trained clients with scoliosis.

In my younger life I was a cardiac nurse and, building on this knowledge, have over the past 14 years been qualified as a cardiac rehab exercise specialist and started the cardiac rehabilitation programme at Aspire.

When I was still working as a cardiac nurse I was diagnosed with multiple sclerosis (MS). I suffered numbness throughout my body. It took some time to get over this attack and on recovery I wanted to start exercising. This was 30 years ago and there were no books about exercising with MS and the doctors did not seem to know much about it either! This life shock was the reason I decided to become a personal trainer specialising in disabled people, hence I started working for Aspire. I wanted to help people who had suffered as I had, with informed advice on how to exercise safely and effectively with their disability and reach their full potential.

During my time at Aspire I came across many patients from the Royal National Orthopaedic Hospital who had not only cardiac problems but also scoliosis. I found myself struggling to construct a training programme without having knowledge as to what would be safe for someone who had had scoliosis surgery.

When I met Caroline Freedman, who was an experienced trainer specialising in scoliosis, I encouraged her to write this book because I felt there was a need for an informed practical guide regarding exercise with scoliosis. Caroline has scoliosis herself and is also an experienced personal trainer with more than 22 years' experience. She has had the condition since she was 15, and has had three major spinal operations. With exercising she has managed to alleviate pain, build up strength and flexibility, improve her posture, gain a good cardiovascular fitness and, all in all, is a remarkable woman and role model. I knew when I met her there was a real need for this book and she was the person who was very capable of producing it based upon her own experience.

This book is both informative and easy to follow. It addresses all facets of fitness for someone with scoliosis. There are well illustrated exercises for strength training, flexibility, body-muscle balance and the cardiovascular component of fitness. These exercises have been tried and tested by Caroline and her many clients, with excellent results. There is a section of 'Dos and Don'ts' which is excellent, ensuring that the client exercises in a way that is not only effective but safe. There is also a section on lifestyle. This includes suggestions regarding clothing and footwear together with other practical matters – for example, positioning pillows when lying down to exercise and to sleep, etc. Advice is given on sports that are beneficial and those which are better avoided as they may be detrimental to people with this condition.

Without reservation, I highly recommend this book, and the writer. I will be using it in the Aspire gym and recommending it to my colleagues. I am very proud of Caroline and her journey to where she is today. She is an inspiration to anyone with scoliosis. This book will help others with general spinal problems too.

Foreword by Zeinab Choudray – a client (aged 29)

I really think this guide is brilliant and will be a huge success and a help to many people.

I started training with Caroline in 2017 after I had experienced a string of health issues. I have a rare brittle bone condition known as *osteogenesis imperfecta* which is further compounded by my scoliosis. After having my spine fused in 2005 when I was just 16 years old, I tried multiple physios and hydrotherapy with some success; however, I never thought it would be possible for me to train like my friends and family – but I was wrong.

I was drawn to Caroline due to her personal experience with scoliosis. She took the time to get to know my limitations due to my extensive hip and femoral surgeries as well as my scoliosis. She showed me how to exercise in a way that would not put further strain on my spine and hips and, even better, showed me numerous exercises that helped me stretch my back and release the tension that was building – downward-facing dog (page 71), pelvic tilt (page 58) and the banister stretch (page 111) are my all-time favourites!

If I'm ever in a situation where my back is playing up and I need someone to speak to, I know Caroline has a wealth of knowledge to tap into – from my desperate 2 a.m. texts from hospital, to me complaining in our PT sessions, she manages to find something to take the edge off and relieve some of the pressure. I am confident the readers of this guide will find the exercises and tips as helpful as I have.

Zeinab

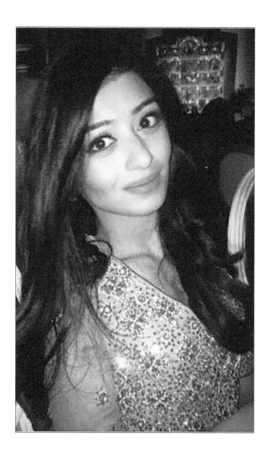

INTRODUCTION

S

My scoliosis journey

Let's start with my credibility to advise anyone with scoliosis how to exercise safely, effectively and efficiently. I have been a busy personal trainer for 22 years. During that time I have come across both children and adults with scoliosis – pre surgery and post surgery, brace believers and wearers and non brace believers, people who are not so affected by scoliosis and others who are terribly self-conscious and frightened.

My scoliosis was discovered in an exercise class when I was 15 years old, by my best friend and her mother, who was the instructor. I was doing a back stretch at the end of a class – hands on the bar, bent over, knees slightly bent, flat back... only mine wasn't.

My mother had always told me not to be so round shouldered and to stand up straight. I used to practise walking round the house with a book on my head! I had complained of a slight pulling feeling of my ribs on my right-hand side for a while. Once my parents had received a call from my friend's mother, I was dragged straight down to our GP. He looked at my spine, made me touch my toes and from then on we were launched into the minefield of scoliosis and began to discover how it would change the direction of my life.

Advised to exercise, I took those sound words to heart and have exercised ever since. My curve was already over 56 degrees and it was just a case of management to prevent surgery for as long as possible so I could finish growing.

I had two main interests in life – acting, which my parents were against, and sewing. I was accepted to four drama schools and also to London College of Fashion. A term into my Design and Pattern Cutting course and my spine had decided to fall like a tree – a double curve of 76 and 82 degrees.

The centre of my ribs was under my left breast. My rib cage was humped on the right side of my back. My heart and lungs were being crushed.

I have had three scoliosis and rib correction surgeries:

1987 – aged 20

1989 – aged 23

2015 – aged 49

Surgery 1

Spinal fusion (thoracic) T2–T11

Harrington rod entire length of spine.

Five ribs cut off on right-hand side and used for bone grafts. Wore a brace for six months.

Beautiful thin scar.

Surgery 2

Harrington rod snapped in half – the result of my attempting a backbend from standing.

Obvious tip: Never do this - I was an idiot!

One fusion hadn't quite taken and so that is where my rod snapped.

Long rod taken out and two shorter rods inserted each side of my thoracic spine. Another rib taken out.

Wore a brace for six months.

Thin but double scar.

Surgery 3

My curve was the same and fused but my spine had decided to rotate and so I had 'shark back' (transverse processes – the little side bones of the spine – were sticking out). This meant that sitting on a high-back chair or lying on a flat surface was very uncomfortable. The skin was also super-sensitive as the metal from one rod was slightly protruding and very near the surface of my skin. I also had two lower ribs on my right-hand side sticking out, so when I tried to lie down or do abdominal crunches all the pressure and weight of my body was on those two ribs, making the skin sore.

I had walked around like this for years and finally – after chickening out and cancelling my surgeries twice – I became so fed up that I just went for it and took the final road to my correction.

One rod was removed and the other shaved at each end. It was too embedded in my spine to be removed. My bottom two ribs on the right-hand side were removed. (They won't grow back, so I didn't need to wear a brace. Yes, that's seven ribs gone altogether.)

Double scar cut out and replaced with a new scar.

I woke up in the High Dependency Unit and couldn't believe my luck – for the first time ever, I was lying flat and could actually feel the left side of my back. Wow, wow, wow. I can't tell you how that moment felt. It wasn't until after several months following my recovery that I realised just how uncomfortable I had been every day.

My quality of life is incredibly improved. I can sit in most chairs. I can lie flat in bed. My back is not as sensitive. I can do small crunches! I can even travel Economy on a flight longer than three hours. Before, having to sit on an airline seat with no room to sit any other way except bolt upright with a body that just did not conform to the ergonomics of airline chairs meant that after three hours I would have searing pain down my legs and a very sore lower and upper spine, and end up in silent tears. Unless I had enough money/miles to upgrade to Business, I wouldn't travel further than Spain.

Below is a quote from the email I sent to my surgeon's secretary from my holiday. I'm not sure how many people would be so excited to sit in Economy:

Also please tell him that I sat for five hours in economy on a plane yesterday! No room for an upgrade and my back feels nothing! So happy – normally I would be so sore. Also lay flat on a bed in the sun today and not sore.

That was my scoliosis journey.

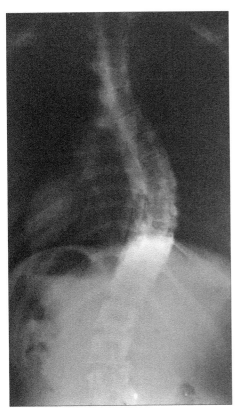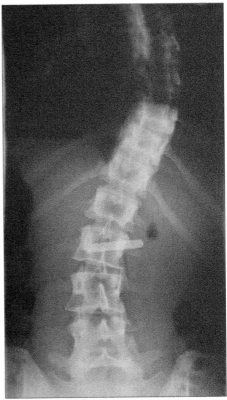

These two X-rays show images of my spine and ribs. Note how my ribs are off centre, creating my rib hump. These are the last X-rays I can find of my spine before surgery. My spinal curve progressed quite rapidly from the decision to operate at a consultation in November 1986 up until January 1987 when I had scoliosis and rib correction surgery.

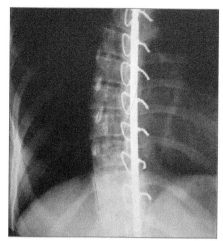 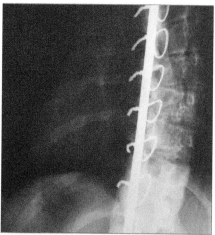

First Surgery. I'm straight. X-rays of my spine taken after surgery
in January 1987. Five ribs have been removed
from my right hand side.

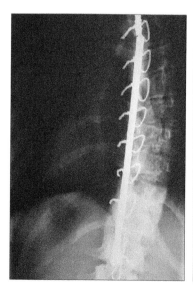 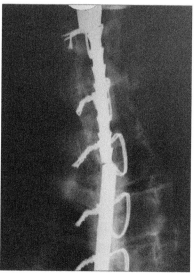

Snapped rod. X-rays of my spine taken in November 1989. Look
closely and you can see where it has broken, approximately ¼
from the top of the rod.

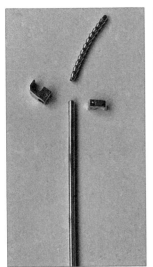
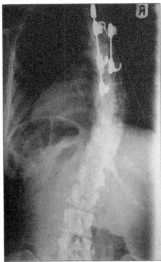

Second Surgery. November 1989. The rod is out. Mr Edgar, my surgeon gave the parts to me as a souvenir. You can see the snapped rod in two pieces and two of the bolts used to attach the rod to the spine. X-ray of my spine after the second surgery in November 1989, showing two rods. The long Harrington rod has been removed and replaced with two shorter rods. This X-ray was taken in June 1991.

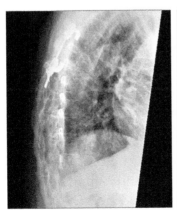
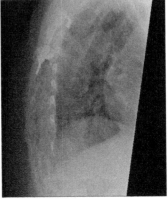

Third Surgery. September 2015. Lateral View. One rod has been taken out, the other shaved down. Two lower ribs removed from my right hand side.

How I became a personal trainer

On balance, personal training is probably not the first choice career for someone with scoliosis. However, it could be said that I, more than most trainers, have the added advantage of not only a working knowledge through years of experience of training clients with this condition, but also had at some point most of the feelings, thoughts and fears my clients have had. I know what that 'pulling' sensation feels like – the one you get across the back of your ribs on the side of your hump before surgery. Also, the panic of walking into a restaurant and knowing the shape of the chairs is going to make you suffer tomorrow and probably the day after too. I know how it feels to do a stomach crunch and have sore ribs where your hump is.

I wanted to have children and was told by my surgeon I would have to be incredibly fit to get through pregnancy without backache and putting a strain on my spine.

I had exercised since I was 14, so I wasn't completely out of shape and had worked out regularly in a gym at least three times a week to keep my back strong. However, I needed to take it up a notch and so I decided I needed a personal trainer. Twenty-seven years ago the fitness industry was just starting to explode. There was only one trainer at my gym who I wanted to use. She was absolutely spot-on with her training and technique. I used to go to Lotte Berk classes (similar to barre), where my scoliosis was discovered, and it was easy to see that the trainer I wanted was on another level of expertise compared with other trainers.

The problem was she didn't want me as a client. She hadn't heard of scoliosis and when I told her the details – fusions, nuts, bolts, wires, screws, rods plus rib removal and a nice long scar – she said 'No way!' Every time I saw her training someone, I would tell her she was going to train me one day and it became a bit of a joke between us. Then one day she approached me. She said she would take me on if I would explain everything about scoliosis to her and what I could and couldn't do. What had changed her mind? She had been asked to train four young girls, one of whom had had scoliosis surgery and was struggling with some of the moves raising her arms, and her back was aching.

I started a training program with the trainer two to three times a week and did another two sessions on my own in the gym. By the time I was pregnant I was super strong and didn't have a day's backache. I continued working out through my pregnancy. My physio at the time insisted that I work my stomach muscles hard to support my extra load. I kept up with the same intensive workouts – lunges, squats, bent-arm pullovers, seated row, crunches – throughout my second pregnancy too.

By that time my trainer had been approached by *GMTV*/*This Morning* to be their fitness guru. She was writing for publications too and was cutting back on her availability for personal training sessions. She was the one who suggested I should qualify as a trainer. At first I thought she had lost the plot. At the time, I was working as a freelance fashion stylist. The more I thought about it, however, and with her encouragement, I realised I had so much knowledge of spinal issues that I could use it to really help other people with similar problems. Exercise has always taken my pain away. If I don't work out for a couple of weeks, my back feels it.

So I enrolled at the London Central YMCA to train in weights and circuits. Worried that I would not be able to keep up with the other people on the course, I was really nervous. I needn't have been. I was the strongest woman and could outdo most of the men on circuits.

Thanks to my amazing trainer, I qualified and have had a 22-year career in an industry I love.

My personal trainer was the brave and lovely Nicki Waterman who sadly passed away in 2016.

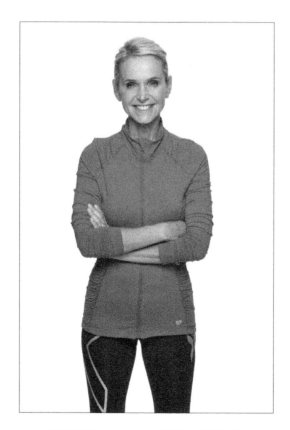

Nicki Waterman (1964–2016),
my personal trainer courtesy of Stewart Williams

Zoe's scoliosis story

Zoe Gibber is my daughter.

Scoliosis can be genetic. I was told when I fell pregnant in the 1990s that one in five children from parents with scoliosis will have some form of curvature. Research since has flagged up various theories, the most recent being that it can be as a result of diet, possibly lack of meat. I am a nutritional advisor but I am not qualified to comment, except to say that I do not advocate fad diets. I am also not convinced that a pure vegan diet can benefit a growing child.

Both my babies had their spines checked in the womb by Kyprianos 'Kypros' Nicolaides, the world-renowned specialist in fetal medicine, and then by an orthopaedic consultant at each milestone – sitting, crawling, walking – and then every few years. I was constantly scanning their spines. When Zoe was 15, I noticed that a slight curvature had developed.

She saw three surgeons for an opinion. The first diagnosed one leg shorter than the other and suggested a leg lift in her shoe. I wasn't convinced and took Zoe to my physiotherapist, John Rutherford. He re-aligned her spine. Both legs were now the same length and he too was convinced Zoe had scoliosis.

We visited another consultant. He diagnosed scoliosis and was amazed I had spotted it as it was only 28 degrees and hard to see without an X-ray. The subject of a brace was introduced and Zoe was really not happy. She persuaded me to take her to a third consultant. He agreed that bracing was needed and explained that, as Zoe was at the end of her adolescence and had nearly stopped growing, it would be an ideal time to do this and she had a very good prognosis for a positive outcome. (X-rays of the wrist can show when the bones stop growing.)

Watching your child being fitted for a brace is not an easy moment. Persuading a self-conscious teenager to walk around with a massive plastic corset is a huge challenge. She didn't want to tell her friends. When they found out they were immensely supportive. The boys at her school nagged her to wear it. So between all of us, she did, although mostly at night instead of daytime, for six months.

The result? Zoe's scoliosis reduced from a 28-degree thoracic curvature to 18 degrees, then settled and naturally fused at 22 degrees. I am immensely grateful, proud and relieved that Zoe agreed to wear her brace.

Hello, my name is Zoe and I'm 24 and scoliosis free.

When I was 15 I was told that I had scoliosis and enough of a curvature of my spine to wear a back brace — not exactly ideal when you're in school. I was really upset about having to wear a brace, embarrassed and worried about what my friends or other people in my year would think as I didn't know anyone else with the same problem.

At first I was angry and hardly wore it, but then I realised if I just sucked it up and didn't care what people thought, I would have a straight back and the chore of wearing an uncomfortable, thick, plastic bodice would soon be over.

So I wore it every night and as much in the day as I could, because I knew that dealing with my scoliosis was exactly what I needed to do to get rid of it.

The brace really helped me and I hope anyone reading this who is in my position understands that your health is the most important thing and choosing to wear a brace over having a curved spine is a no-brainer. I'm happy I dealt with my back properly as I am now practically straight. It was definitely worth it and I urge anyone in my position to do the same.

Zoe Gibber

What is Scoliosis?

At its simplest, scoliosis is an abnormal curvature of the spine. There are four common types:

• Right thoracic curve – curve to the right (thoracic) upper back.

• Right thoracolumbar curve – curve bends to the right of the thoracic down to the lumbar (lower back).

• Right lumbar curve – curve bends to the right of the lumbar.

• Double major curve – usually a curve to the right at the thoracic and left at the lumbar.

Diagnosis includes bending over to touch the toes and checking to see how symmetrical the spine appears plus X-ray, CT scan and MRI.

Signs of scoliosis as advised by the NHS include:

• A visibly curved spine

• Leaning to one side

• Uneven shoulders

• One shoulder or hip sticking out

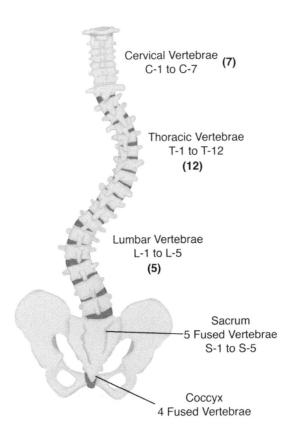

Cervical Vertebrae
C-1 to C-7 **(7)**

Thoracic Vertebrae
T-1 to T-12
(12)

Lumbar Vertebrae
L-1 to L-5
(5)

Sacrum
5 Fused Vertebrae
S-1 to S-5

Coccyx
4 Fused Vertebrae

• The ribs sticking out on one side

• Clothes not fitting well

• Some back pain.

(Reference: www.nhs.uk/conditions/scoliosis/)To provide more detail I have asked the specialist physiotherapist John Rutherford MSCP DC HCPC, to describe the key aspects and background of the condition. John is my physiotherapist. Twelve years ago, I was in dreadful pain and a surgeon referred me to him. John realigned my hips and right shoulder and his method of working continues to relieve any of the pains I sometimes get. He is not called 'the miracle worker' by his patients for nothing (as overheard many times in the waiting room at his clinic).

An introduction to scoliosis
By John Rutherford MCSP DC HCPC

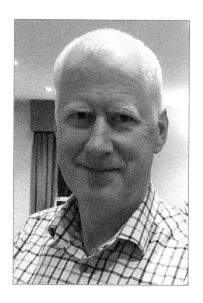

Introduction

I have known and treated Caroline for many years following her spinal fusion. I'm delighted I have been able to provide treatment which has made a positive contribution to her health and life. Having reviewed her book on exercise for scoliosis, I was delighted to be asked to contribute this introductory section. This book will be a useful and practical guide for those who are able to exercise to alleviate the postural and funtional bias of their scoliosis curves, and also for those who need a more radical solution, and require detailed exercise guidance following surgery.

John Rutherford: www.backpainspecialistslondon.co.uk

Scoliosis

Scoliosis is a three-dimensional spinal deformity, focused in the middle and lower spine. The normal curves of the spine are distorted from front to back, side to side, and rotated. There is a genetic factor involved in many cases of scoliosis.

A scoliosis curve is commonly 'S' shaped, with a rib hump lifting the shoulder blade, uneven shoulder height and frontal rib and waist folds.

Parents with scoliosis, or a family history, should carefully observe their children for developing curves.

CONTRIBUTORY FACTORS TO IDIOPATHIC SCOLIOSIS

In idiopathic (of unknown cause) scoliosis, a genetic factor is thought not to be the only cause. Current research has identified other contributory factors. These include imbalance of growth hormones that may affect bone density and cartilage development. Oestrogen blood levels have an influence on normal bone formation. Calmodulin, a calcium-binding receptor protein, regulates platelets and the contractile properties of muscles.

Altered levels of blood platelets have been observed. Collagen and elastin fibres are the base elements of the supporting ligaments and discs of the spine. Structural abnormalities have been observed in discs and ligaments in individuals with progressive spinal curves. There is also evidence that the spinal curves may be due to an imbalance in neurotransmitters.

NEUROTRANSMITTERS

Neurotransmitter testing for scoliosis is vital and can help pinpoint a serious deficiency in serotonin, which can influence spine curvature. Neurotransmitters are chemicals that carry messages from the brain, via the nerves, to muscles, prompting the spine to make adjustments in response to external changes. Postural control centres are located in the hind brain, the area of the brain that is located in the rear and lower region, and are not under voluntary control. Epinephrine, formed in the adrenal glands on top of the kidneys (it helps the body to adapt to sudden changes), and serotonin are neurotransmitters, formed from the essential amino acids, tyrosine and tryptophan. The B vitamins assist the synthesis of numerous neurochemical and signalling molecules. These hormones assist neural transmission and help the body to adjust to new and sudden changes in position. Folic acid (vitamin B9) helps maintain normal levels of serotonin. Vitamins B6 and B12 contribute to the myelin sheath around nerve cells, which speeds signals through the brain. Studies indicate that niacin (vitamin B3) helps in the synthesis and repair of DNA, and that it has a role in signalling between nerve cells. The essential nature of these different substances emphasises the importance of good nutrition.

DIET AND NUTRITION

Current research indicates that diet and nutrition can contribute to developing scoliosis. Calcium and vitamin D levels need to be adequate for correct bone density. Correct blood iron levels are essential for normal bone formation and synthesis of connective tissue. Haeme protein in animal-based foods binds larger quantities of iron, aiding absorption in the gut and providing fuel for the muscles. Vegetable-based food lacks the haeme-binding iron protein, rendering iron absorption in the gut less efficient. Poor teenage diets or unmonitored vegan or vegetarian diets can have an impact on normal blood chemistry, affecting bone density in adolescents.

Phytate, a substance found at high levels in soy and many types of beans, legumes and seeds with a high-fibre content, is a strong inhibitor of iron absorption. Research suggests a possible 30% loss of bone density in adolescents with progressive spinal curves.

Some statistics indicate increasing numbers of teenagers and young adults demonstrate thyroid dysfunction. Correct thyroid levels are essential for adequate bone density and structural integrity.

ADOLESCENT IDIOPATHIC SCOLIOSIS

Adolescent idiopathic scoliosis (AIS) forms the bulk of conditions seen in our clinics. As I have said, 'idiopathic' scoliosis describes a spinal curve of unknown cause. This occurs in 2–3% of both sexes between the ages of 10 and 16 years. However, it is up to 10 times more likely that the curve will progress in girls than in boys. Curve progression may be rapid during growth spurts in adolescence. A curve can be easily identified by the trained eye. X-ray or MRI imaging can be helpful in addition. Bone maturity can be observed in the pelvic bones using what is called the 'Reiser grading scale' observed in the bone known as the ilium: grade 1 indicates immature bone, while grade 5 confirms growth plate fusion, allowing no further growth.

COBB ANGLE – THE MEASUREMENT OF THE DEGREE OF SIDE-TO-SIDE SPINAL CURVATURE

The 'Cobb angle' is used to determine the degree of spinal curvature. If the Cobb angle is below 30 degrees at bone maturity, the curve should remain stable. If it is above 30 degrees, the curve may gradually progress through adult life. If the Cobb angle is measured manually, there can be a 5-degree discrepancy in accuracy. Modern software advances should eliminate this.

CLINICAL PRESENTATION

A scoliotic curve is often painless. Pain may come from stress on affected structures. Rapid curve development can be painful, and cause organ compression. Breathing function can be impaired if rib distortion impacts on the lungs.

Scoliosis in a newborn child or observed in a child under the age of 10 years may have a genetic origin. Spina bifida is a possible cause of scoliosis. Scientists suspect the factors that cause spina bifida are multiple: genetic, nutritional and environmental. Research indicates a lack of folic acid in the mother's diet is a key factor. A child with acquired cerebral palsy, a group of permanent movement disorders that appear in early childhood, may develop infantile scoliosis.

STRUCTURAL VERSUS FUNCTIONAL CURVES

Idiopathic scoliosis accounts for 70–90% of all scoliosis. A structural scoliosis is fixed and cannot be altered by position or manipulation. Clinical examination will often reveal that a scoliosis that appears to be idiopathic and structural is, in fact, a functional curve (caused by defective movement or position). A structural curve will not release with forward bending of the body. However, a functional curve often corrects when testing body positions. Functional curves can be caused by altered spine, pelvic and sacrum alignment, leg length differences, poor posture, muscle tightness, weakness and altered head and neck position. Defective alignment of the head with the neck, or a 'subluxed' (loss of normal alignment) position of the neck vertebrae, particularly the 1st and 2nd segments, can be contributory factors.

DEGENERATIVE CURVES

A degenerative curve in adults is caused by progressive joint damage to the spinal segments, falling bone density and weakening of muscle. It presents as a C-shaped curve. It usually affects those above the age of 50. Falling hormone levels (i.e. oestrogen in women), and nutritional deficiencies, contribute to lower bone density. A number of people lose the ability to absorb and maintain adequate vitamin B12 and folate levels. Flat feet, decreased levels of exercise and less effective body balance contribute to curve formation.

TREATMENT

Any treatment for scoliosis requires a full and precise understanding of the type of scoliosis under observation. When a spine is tested in a neutral position, vertebrae with a concave bend to the left will bend to the left but rotate to the right. In a non-neutral spine, such as forward bending with a concavity to the left, vertebrae will bend to the left and rotate to the left also. The alternative occurs if the concavity occurs to the right.

It is essential to understand the joint and muscle positions to deliver correct manual corrections. Muscle on one aspect of a curve will be contracted and 'weak', the opposite stretched and 'weak'. The decisions to be made are which to strengthen and which to stretch. Treatment of scoliosis in a child pre-puberty requires a paediatrician.

Functional and degenerative scoliosis can be treated with manual techniques derived from physiotherapy, osteopathy and chiropractic. This would include correction of vertebral position, stretching and strengthening of muscles, and functional exercise to retrain and reinforce body balance through the brain–nerve–muscle pathways.

Surgical intervention may be required if exercise and bracing can't modify curve progression. Bracing and activity suits can be most useful in curves below 30° in an adolescent approaching bone maturity (Reiser grade 4–5). It is possible to correct any unfused segments following surgery to improve body alignment.

It is relatively easy and inexpensive for parents, care workers and GPs to learn how to observe potential scoliosis. Observation is key to early intervention and early treatment is more effective than later.

Parents can observe a curve in a small child with minimal prompting. A teacher may notice a curve in PE. A GP may observe this during an examination for another issue. It is feasible to test for scoliosis, particularly AIS, in less than one minute. There is a simple forward-bending test.

Correct levels of exercise, tailored to the age group, are essential in dealing with any spinal curve. In adolescents, too much exercise can often be as detrimental as too little. Poor posture must be corrected. Diet and blood chemistry need to be evaluated and adjusted if indicated. Any exercise program should address correct body balance.

TERMINOLOGY

Abductors muscles in the outer thighs.

Abs abdominals – stomach muscles.

Adductors muscles in the inner thighs.

Alignment (body alignment) – how the head, shoulders, spine, hips, knees and toes line up with each other.

Bi's biceps – muscles in the front of the upper arms.

Bracs brachialis and brachioradialis – upper arm muscles lying deeper than the biceps – also used in pulling a rowing cable.

Cervical spine top of the spine – neck – made up of seven vertebrae (C1: Atlas), (C2: Axis) through C7; this is concave posterior (backwards).

Congenital scoliosis Curvature of the spine from birth.

Costoplasty or thoracoplasty Procedure of rib removal for those suffering from a rib hump.

Coccyx the 'tailbone'.

Core a term describing the abs, lats, chest musculature, pelvic and back muscles – the trunk.

Crunch abdominal exercise where the lower back stays on the floor, the pelvis is tilted upwards and the head and upper body are gently lifted off, with arms supporting the head. The legs are bent and either on the floor or elevated.

Delts posterior deltoids, infraspinatus, and teres minor– shoulder muscles – used in the rowing action.

Discs intervertebral discs – these lie between the vertebrae in the spinal column. If any of these slip out from or protrude between the vertebrae they touch the spinal cord, causing acute pain down the spine, arms and legs. This is a 'slipped disc', a condition separate from scoliosis.

Double curvature where the spine has two abnormal sideways curves making an 'S' shape

Glutes the gluteus maximus, gluteus medius and gluteus minimus muscles – the buttocks.

Hamstrings a group of three muscles and their tendons located at back of the upper leg, from the hip to the knee, used for walking and running.

Hip flexors (Iliopsoas) muscles that bring legs and trunk together.

Idiopathic scoliosis curvature of the spine of unknown cause thought to happen during puberty and onwards.

Isometric a static (not moving) contraction of a muscle without any movement of the muscle or related joint.

Lats latissimus dorsi – the large broad muscles that you can feel stretching by touching your left upper back with your right hand – used to bring the arms towards the rowing machine.

Lumbar spine lower part of the spine around the waist – made up of five vertebrae L1–L5; this is concave.

Lunges exercise that works the quadraceps (front leg muscles) and glutes (bottom) by stepping forward and bending the front and back leg.

Obliques part of the group of abdominal muscles – used for side bending and rotation.

Pecs pectoralis or chest muscles; move the shoulder joint.

Pelvic floor exercises Muscles around uterus, bladder, bowel and vagina/penis. To find them, pretend you are urinating, tighten muscles drawing in and tightening. With anal muscle, tighten the area as if avoiding passing wind, then relax.

Pelvis Lower part of trunk of body, including hips. Protects internal organs and bears weight of upper body when sitting/standing.

Plank	isometric (static) position where the body faces downwards on the floor in a push-up with the forearms resting on the floor.
Rhoms	rhomboids – muscles that support the upper back (the part of your upper back that's tough to reach, especially when it's itchy!) – used to retract the scapular (shoulder blades).
Quads	quadriceps – muscles in the front of the thighs.
Sacral spine	very bottom of the spine – convex.
Sit ups	abdominal exercise where the entire spine comes off the floor. It puts stress on the spine and neck. Please do not ever attempt this. I do not give these to any clients.
Spinal fusion	surgery to connect two or more vertebrae together, creating solid bone with no movement or space.
Spinal muscles	erector spinae – muscles that support the spine – used to keep your body upright.
Squats	strength exercise for the lower body. Lower hips from standing position and stand back up. This works the quads (thighs), glutes (bottom), adductor (inner thigh) and hamstring muscles. The squat also isometrically (static) uses the erector spinae and abdominal muscles.
Thoracic spine	upper back portion of the spine where the ribs are located – made up of 12 vertebrae T1–T12; this is convex.
Transverse processes	small, irregular-shaped boney structures that protrude outwards from the sides of the vertebrae (spine).
Traps	Traps – trapezius – the triangular muscles located from base of head, neck and across thoracic area (upper back). Helps neck, shoulders and arms move.
Tri's	triceps – muscles in the back lower part of the upper arms.
Vertebrae	Vertebrae – run from head to tailbone, 33 segments of the spinal column (7 cervical, 12 thoracic, 5 lumbar, 5 sacral, 4 coccygeal vertebrae) 24 move.

GETTING STARTED

I am presuming you want to feel better than you do right now and also look better.

I am not a surgeon or a physiotherapist and this guide is not intended to contradict anything you may have been advised to do/not do. The following Dos and Don'ts come from my experience as both a scoliosis patient and a personal trainer who has years of experience working with scoliosis clients. Some of those clients have had surgery and others have not.

I am convinced, through research and both personal and professional involvement with scoliosis, that strong muscles around the spine directly contribute to a reduction in pain. That is my experience and that of my clients.

I was asked to write guidelines for exercising with scoliosis by Liz Bord – the head physiotherapist at the Royal National Orthopaedic Hospital, Stanmore for their Aspire Leisure Centre Gym. This was because many people are not told what they can and cannot do after surgery. Either they avoid exercise, or they go to classes where the instructor has no knowledge of scoliosis and they end up totally confused as to what will be okay for them.

The following chapters are for physiotherapists as well as for personal trainers and scoliosis patients. This is meant as a flick-through, easy, dip-in-and-dip-out guide.

Please always consult a health professional to check that any of these Dos, Don'ts and Tips are safe for you individually.

PART 1

EXERCISE BEFORE SCOLIOSIS SURGERY

Regular exercise will really help to stretch and strengthen the muscles around your spine, keeping them strong. As a result, posture will improve and you will look and feel so much better. There is no reason why anyone with scoliosis who has not had surgery should be restricted in any way with exercise and so there are not many exercises or activities to avoid. It is a case of listening to recommendations from the consultant, physiotherapist and your body as to what may be comfortable to do. The exercises I have recommended for post scoliosis surgery are also good for strengthening your body generally while living your day-to-day life with scoliosis. So do look at those too (see page 51). The general rule for any exercise program is that if it hurts, stop, or change position.

There are different schools of thought about whether working out one side of the opposing curve of the spine, more than the other, will help to both stabilise and prevent the spine from curving further. Exercise does not prevent scoliosis but it does help with pain, posture, strength, stamina and wellbeing.

Before I had my third surgery my back looked uneven. I tried doing more repetitions on the weaker-looking side of my back to build up the lat muscle (see page 27). I used the lat pulldown machine (see page 76) to do this, with the lightest possible weight on the machine, and performed double the number of repetitions using just my left arm (my weaker side). I then used both my arms to perform more sets of the exercise. After two months my back did look a little more symmetrical due to the build-up of muscle on my left side and I felt stronger. I often apply this method to scoliosis clients to help strengthen their bodies.

Many children and adults who suffer from mild scoliosis through to more severe can feel some level of pain at any point during their lives. A 'pulling' sensation across the ribs where the muscles are stretched over the rib hump is often described to me by my scoliosis clients. I also felt the 'pulling' sensation before my first surgery. I agree with the professional opinion that exercise helps with pain and not only experienced this myself but my scoliosis clients have all reported back to me that their pain levels decreased.

I was advised by my consultant, Mr Michael Edgar, to get super strong before my surgery. I worked out with free weights, resistance machines and body weight. I also attended a variety of fitness classes. It is widely recognised that the fitter you are before surgery, the quicker your full recovery will be. Exercises in the Dos After Scoliosis Surgery chapter (page 51) can also be used for rehabilitation.

DO:

- Exercise as much as you can.

- Keep up with seeing a physiotherapist.

- Keep your back strong.

- If you feel it will help your pain, try having a massage from someone who really knows what they are doing. Research your therapist. Don't be scared to walk away from someone you feel will do more harm than good.

- If your ribs are very uneven and it is not comfortable to lie flat on the floor, take a small cushion, a wedge or even a soft hoodie to balance your body evenly on the floor. Play around with your positioning to make yourself comfortable.

- Avoid any exercise where you have to put your body further out of alignment.

- Use the mirrors in the gym if you are exercising on your own to check your positioning.

- Be very careful when performing abdominal exercises to keep your legs high so as not to place any extra pressure on your spine.

I asked personal trainer Julia Blass, who has worked in the exercise industry for over 30 years, for her tips on living with scoliosis and what to do before surgery or if surgery may not be needed. She has scoliosis, but has not had surgery. She is a huge fan of the roller which can be used for pain relief as a massage tool if there are no fusions or rods.

Julia recommends the following for her scoliosis clients:

- rolling from upper to lower spine on your back.
- massaging your hips, lying on your side and rolling back and forth.
- massaging your buttocks by sitting on the roller and moving back and forth.
- lying on your front and massaging your quads back and forth.
- massaging your calves by sitting with your ankles in front on top of the roller and moving them back and forth.

Julia recommends spinal twisting to loosen up the back – with direction from your physio or personal trainer.

TP TRIGGER POINT THERAPY BALL

Again, always check with your physiotherapist.

Julia is a huge fan of these balls. She says they have directly eased the pulling and pain in her back that she gets from her scoliosis.

She uses them to provide direct deep tissue compression similar to a therapist applying pressure during remedial massage.

- Stand against a wall and place the ball where your pain is.
- Roll the ball up and down.

Julia says, 'It will be painful but then, like magic, you will feel a release of the pain as the muscle relaxes from spasm.'

PART 2

THE DON'Ts AFTER SCOLIOSIS SURGERY

Here is a selection of exercises to be avoided or limited if you have had scoliosis surgery.

✖ BACK BENDS

NEVER – and there are no alternatives.

Often practised in yoga, etc.

These are a very bad idea if the spine is fused with rods. This is one of the reasons my first Harrington rod snapped.

✖ SHOULDER STAND

NEVER – no alternatives.

This curves the spine, puts pressure on metal work and fusion and too much pressure on the upper spine, shoulder blades and shoulders. Nothing beneficial will result from performing this.

✖ HEAD STAND

NEVER – no discussion, no advice, no alternatives.

Shoulder stand

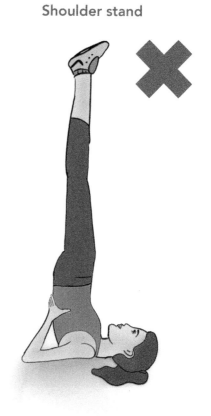

✖ FULL NECK ROLLS

NEVER – no discussion, no advice, no alternatives.

Why? Often T1 (the first thoracic vertebra, at the top of the back) is the only vertebra moving and it puts too much stress on the disc. Neck rolls have been out of fashion for a long time for anyone with or without spinal issues due to the possible injuries to the associated muscles, tendons and vertebrae. If you go to a class where the trainer is demonstrating these, walk out!

✖ SLAM BAGS

These heavy weighted bags to be picked up and slammed down are used in slam classes and circuit workouts. They are too violent and may cause a reverberation through the body.

✖ SPINNING BIKES AND BIKES

These will not necessarily cause damage but the instability of the hips when cycling can cause lower back pain and also hip pain, so I generally avoid them. Also, the positioning of the handle bars often causes strain and pain around the neck and shoulder area. Use with caution after full recovery.

With road cycling, the uneven surface may jar the back. I just do not recommend it.

✖ SHOULDER PRESS – USING FREE WEIGHTS

A huge NO! (see machine shoulder press, page 42)

Abdominal exercises to avoid

✖ SIT UPS

Sit ups are no good for anyone in my opinion. Even a person with a 'normal' spine will start to use their back muscles once they go past a certain point within their spinal range, putting stress on vertebrae and hip flexors.

Never perform an abdominal exercise without supporting your head. The strain on your neck may result in considerable pain in your neck and shoulders.

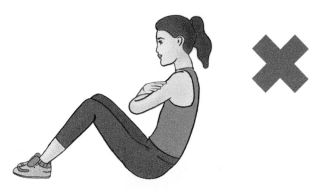

✖ ABDOMINAL EXERCISES INVOLVING LOW LEG LIFTS FROM THE FLOOR

Why not do these? They involve too much stress on the lower back and the risk of arching the spine, which could seriously damage the vertebrae.

✖ ABDOMINAL EXERCISES INVOLVING FRONT TWISTING ROTATIONAL MOVEMENT OR ANY ROTATIONAL SWINGING

Why avoid these? These involve too much pressure on the lower spine. Post surgery, you no longer have a natural curve that bends. The spine will over-compensate and over-use the areas where movement is free, putting immense pressure on those vertebrae. Your remaining moveable vertebrae need to be looked after. I believe that over-movement may contribute to premature degenerative damage to them. Often there is wear and tear to the vertebrae as we age. With scoliosis, those vertebrae that still have movement can be subject to over-compensation, resulting in early wear and tear. The last thing anyone with scoliosis needs is to have further surgery - for example, a cage and more fusions.

The spine should not be arched.

✖ OTHER ABDOMINAL EXERCISES TO AVOID

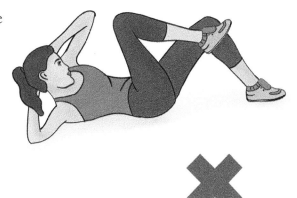

- Diagonal crunches
- Twisting or rotating the body (Russian twists)
- Diagonal crunches with alternate leg lifts criss-crossing legs in the air
- Crunches without support for the head
- Full crunches
- Lifting the legs up from the floor
- Lowering the legs from 90° above the head to the floor to past 30° or 2 pm on the clock when performing lower abdominal exercises
- Taking the arms away from supporting the head
- Using any extra free weights to make an abdominal exercise more difficult
- Arching the spine.

Machine exercises to avoid

✖ WAIST ROTATION MACHINE

Another NO!

Fusion of the spine does not allow complete rotation to each side. There is a danger to swinging from side to side. There are more effective exercises for the obliques (see pages 66-68 and page 92).

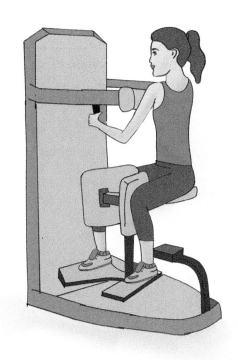

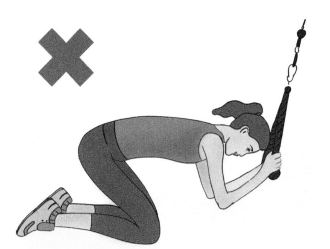

✖ KNEELING ABDOMINAL PULLDOWNS

Avoid – you need a flexible spine to do these, something you do not have!

✖ WEIGHTED ABDOMINAL MACHINE

Avoid this as the weighted load can place too much pressure on your trunk. It is not necessary – there are other exercises that will be more comfortable to do and more effective.

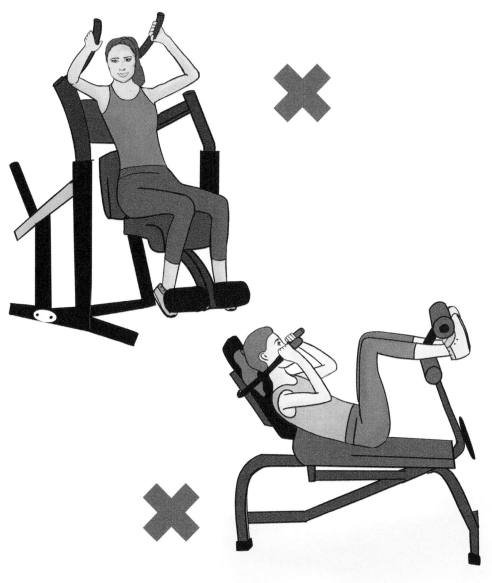

✖ SHOULDER PRESS – USING A MACHINE

A huge NO!

Your configuration is not the same as everyone else's. Accept this. It's never going to work for you. Shoulder presses have to be performed lifting a bar or free weights above your shoulders symmetrically. Scoliosis by its very nature is asymmetrical.

In scoliosis, shoulders are uneven to a greater or lesser degree. The shoulder blade glides over the hump of the rib cage, pushing the shoulder forward. Therefore, the action of a shoulder press exercise and forcing symmetry can push the rest of the back out of alignment.

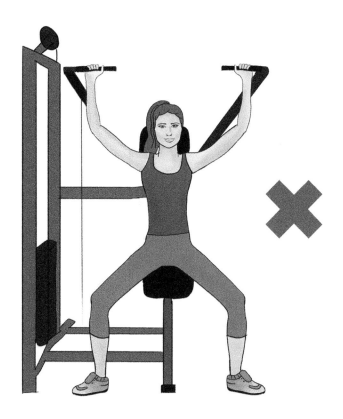

✖ MACHINE DELTOID RAISES – 'ELBOW RAISES'

These will be too heavy before you start.

You will end up very sore.

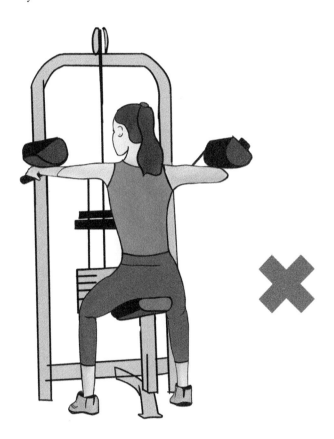

✖ BACK EXERCISE MACHINE

I do not like the look of this machine! I don't use it myself as, in my opinion, there is too much opportunity to strain a muscle. It is akin to picking up a heavy object with a rounded back.

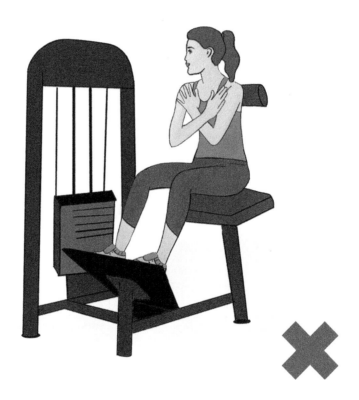

✖ LEG PRESS MACHINE

This compresses the spine when extending both legs. This can put the hips out of alignment when performing with alternate legs.

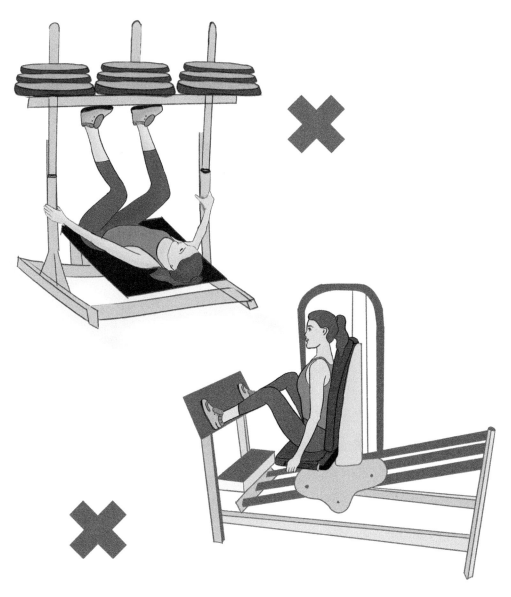

✖ LYING-DOWN LEG CURL MACHINE

This is used to exercise the hamstrings. The positioning of the machine often means that when curling the legs, the pressure is too great on the lower back.

NB: Seated leg curl is okay with a low weight.

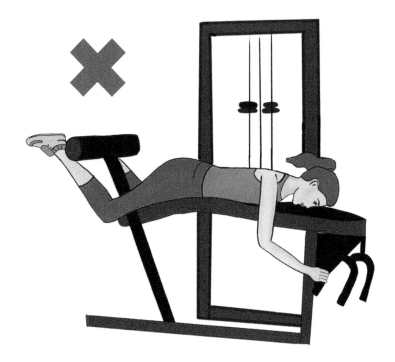

✖ GLUTE MACHINE

NO – it puts a strain on the lower back.

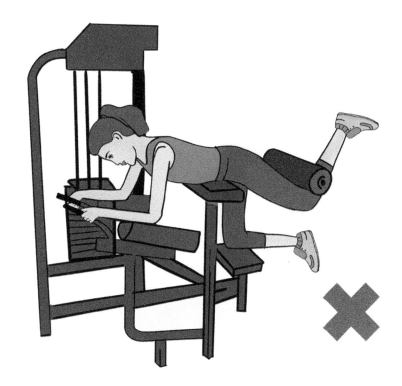

✖ STEPPER

I'm not crazy about these. There is too much opportunity to put the hips out of alignment. However if you do enjoy using this machine avoid long large steps set on a high resistance.

✖ SWISS BALL (see page 101)

The idea of the Swiss ball is working against instability to strengthen the core. While it is great for most people, I do not recommend it for working out with a fused spine in case of twisting the torso while using it. Using the Swiss ball as a seat is fine, but not immediately after surgery. Just wait till you get your balance back. As recovery progresses, John Rutherford advises: 'Supervised exercises on the ball allow more challenging options'.

✖ POWERPLATE, VIBROGYM AND VIBRATION TRAINING MACHINES

Do not use one of these if you have fusions or metal implants in your spine or any other part of the body. It may dislodge the work that has been done.

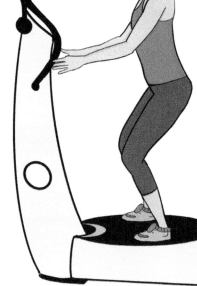

PLEASE NOTE

I love Power Plate, VibroGym and vibration training machines for clients with muscular problems, including MS (multiple sclerosis) and cerebral palsy. I have seen amazing results with some clients over the years. These machines stimulate the muscles, tendons and nerves.

I have witnessed:

1. An MS patient who used a wheelchair at RNOH Aspire Leisure Centre Gym use the Power Plate and for one hour after be able to lift a leg that she had not been able to move for three years.

2. A teenager with cerebral palsy on one side, who had never had any feeling in his hand, place his hand on top of a rubber mat on the PowerPlate for three sets of 60 seconds on Low and say he could feel pins and needles immediately after.

3. Good results with knee injuries when used for strength building.

4. Exceptional muscle strength increase.

But scoliosis is a different matter!

Those are the Don'ts. The good news is that there are lots of Dos and ways to adapt to working out safely and beneficially for your scoliosis.

PART 3

THE DOs
AFTER SCOLIOSIS SURGERY

The idea after scoliosis surgery is to build up back muscles gently.

According to the surgeon from my third surgery, the general rule is to lift no more than 5 kilos with free weights.

Starting back to exercise

PAIN

You should not feel pain during exercise at all. If there is any pain in the joints – back, neck, hips, knees, shoulders, elbows, wrists – stop what you are doing immediately.

Gentle muscle pain after two days is normal in, for example, the quads (thighs), glutes (bottom) and abs (stomach). It is not normal not to be able to walk, or to have terrible neck and shoulder pain or to be in agony. If this happens, either the exercise was performed incorrectly or you have overdone it, or that exercise is definitely not for you.

Do not over-push yourself (or your client) at any time after scoliosis surgery. Initially, fatigue sets in quickly, so always make sure there is a rest time when the session is finished. Chill out for at least 30 minutes afterwards.

With my clients I operate what I call 'exercise allergy awareness':

EXERCISE ALLERGY AWARENESS

- Start with one gentle exercise
- Start with low repetitions
- Wait for two to three days
- If you feel no pain at all after two to three days, continue with the first exercise and add a second
- Wait another two to three days
- If you feel no pain at all, add a third exercise to your routine
- Wait another two to three days
- If you feel no pain at all, add a fourth exercise, and so on ...

If you do feel pain, which at its maximum should be no more than gentle muscle pain, you will now be aware that a particular exercise is to be avoided – just like a food allergy.

POSTURE/ALIGNMENT

At all times be aware of your posture. You (or your client/patient) now have a straighter back. Let's look after it and make the best of the surgical result!

HOW TO STAND AND SIT DURING EXERCISE

This depends on where your fusion (two or more vertebrae joined together) is. Often the vertebrae T1 and above have movement and some parts of your lower spine may also have movement. Always check with the surgeon exactly where there is movement, if any. Also check that all the exercises in this section are safe for you individually to do. I have listed them according to what is suitable for various stages of recovery and beyond. Just be sure to start extremely slowly.

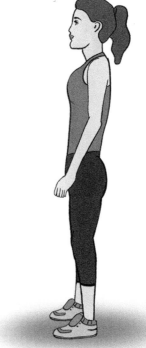

STARTING POSITION

Suck your abs in. Your pelvis should be tilted slightly forward. If you have movement in your lower spine, do not arch it. Shoulders down, head level and chin tucked in. When standing and exercising, always make sure your knees are slightly bent as this will take the pressure off your lower spine. Do not hyperextend (over-straighten) your elbows or knees.

ALIGNMENT

Always be aware of your body alignment. Head, neck, shoulders, spine, hips, knees, ankles and toes should follow each other. A tip is to look down or check yourself in the mirror. Are your knees pulling together or your toes positioned inwards? Your knees should be front facing or slightly outwards and your toes positioned between 11 am and 1 pm OR 10 am and 2 pm.

BREATHING

I find some people concentrate so hard on their exercises that they forget to breathe and hold their breath. Look around any gym and you will probably see someone who is a bit red in the face. In my opinion, the easiest way to get your breathing right while exercising is to:

- Breathe in/inhale through your nose at the easiest point.
- Breathe out/exhale through your mouth at the hardest point (exertion).

Do not hyperventilate and overdo the breathing. It should be gentle or can cause dizziness/light-headedness.

For example, if performing a seated row (see page 80): breathe out as the weight is brought towards your body and in as the weight is released back.

WALKING

Start with walking a few steps, then increase to three minutes and up to 20 minutes per day. Your surgeon should advise you as to how to progress straight after surgery.

Focus on your posture – look in the mirror.

Heel to toe – start walking placing your heel on the floor first, then the middle of your foot, following through with the ball of your foot and finally your toes. Lift your feet when you walk, as opposed to plonking them down or shuffling, not lifting your feet. Be aware of uneven pavements. Keep your shoulders down – your natural protective position may encourage you to close up, with your shoulders up by your ears and slightly forward. Try to nip this postural position in the bud as soon as you can. Open your chest, drop your shoulders, suck in your core. You may feel weird standing upright, as if your body is screaming 'look at me'. You don't look weird? – you're just straighter than you were before your surgery.

SWIMMING

Your surgeon will probably suggest swimming.

It strengthens the entire body. It is good both before and after scoliosis surgery.

Front crawl and backstroke can be a bit of a challenge as often, due to the configuration of your arms, you may go off course in the pool and bump into someone/something.

Breaststroke is easier.

Be careful not to swim with your head in the air.

Floor work

Equipment

Lie on a good quality mat for comfort. For extra comfort at the gym, take your own mat to put over the mats provided.

Also take a small cushion for your head if needed.

A wedge under your glutes and upper thighs supports your lower back and helps you to keep your spine gently pressed into the floor. Roll up a sweatshirt or use a small cushion if you don't have one. Most of the equipment mentioned in this handbook is available from amazon.co.uk, physioroom.com and/or Physicalcompany.co.uk.

Floor work positioning

LYING DOWN ON YOUR BACK

I was always taught to keep my spine glued to the floor. This has prevented me and my clients from having any pain during exercise. There should be as little space as possible between your spine and the floor. Tilt your pelvis and keep your knees bent with your feet flat on the floor, with a wedge under your lower bottom/upper thighs for support. The wedge takes the pressure off your spine.

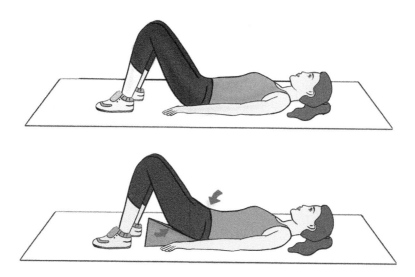

To engage your core, imagine drawing your belly button into your spine, scoop your abdominals in and pull your pelvic floor up. You should feel like everything is being sucked in and your pelvis tilted upwards.

If your hair is tied into a ponytail, make sure it is not interfering with the positioning of your head and neck, e.g. chin tilted too far back or forward. The space between your chin and chest should be about the size of an orange – try using one to gauge where the positioning should be – it works. Remember to breathe, in through your nose and out through your mouth, gently and without hyperventilating, in a relaxed manner.

PELVIC TILT

This exercises your core and pelvic floor muscles:

- Lie on your back

- Knees bent

- Feet hip-width apart.

- Hips, knees, ankles and toes should follow the alignment from your hips. Feet and knees should be slightly turned out – to 11 am and 1 pm or 10 am and 2 pm on the clock.

- Push your spine into the floor and tilt your pelvis up. Do not at this stage lift your pelvis off the floor. Suck your abs in. Squeeze your glutes very gently. (For women, pull in your pelvic floor muscles.) Relax.

- Repeat five times.

- Build up slowly over weeks to 10 x 2 sets.

PELVIC TILT – PROGRESSION OVER TIME

- Lift your hips off the floor.

- Go from flat feet onto tiptoes bringing your feet closer to your bottom.

- Add a Pilates ring or weighted ball (max 3 kg) between your thighs to work the adductors (inside thigh muscles) at the same time.

Start position for pelvic tilt

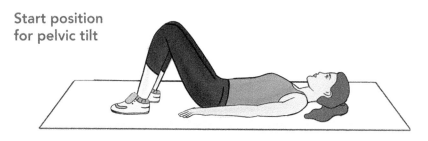

Pelvic tilt

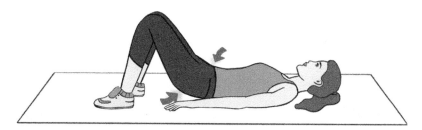

SIDE LEG RAISES

These build strength in hip flexors, glutes, quads (thighs) and abs.

Always have your underneath leg bent for stability and support. Low ankle weights can be added with progression. (Also good for knee injury recovery)

Variations include:

1. Straight upper leg raises.

2. Bending knee in towards the body and out.

3. Top leg parallel with underneath leg – bending the knee gently, bringing the heel back to the glute.

4. Inside thigh – place top leg over lower leg and lift lower leg up.

5. Start with 10 reps on each side, building up to 30 reps x 3 sets.

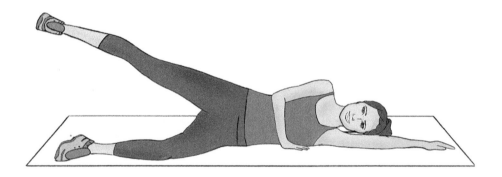

Straight upper leg raises

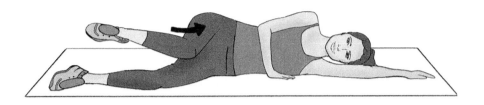

Floorwork quad and glute exercise
Bending knee in towards the body and out

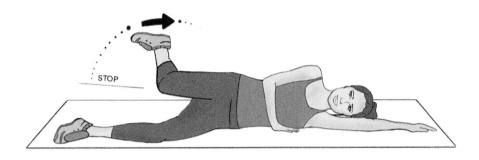

Floorwork hamstring exercise
Top leg parallel with underneath leg – bending the knee gently,
bringing the heel back to the glute

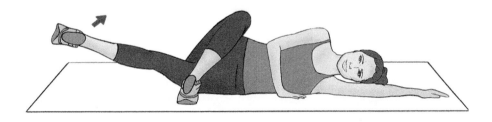

Floorwork inside thigh (adductor) exercise
Inside thigh – place top leg over lower leg and
lift lower leg up

Back strengthening

These exercises strengthen the lats and entire spinal area.

I have listed them in the order to be followed during recovery.

Start with six reps, building up to 20 x 3 sets.

ALTERNATE LEGS

- Start on the floor on all fours
- Suck your stomach in so that your core is solid and fixed
- Do not arch your back
- Slowly extend one leg straight out, hold for as long as is comfortable
- Then repeat on the other side.

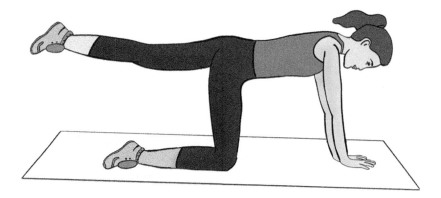

ALTERNATE ARMS

As opposite, with lower legs on the floor, slowly extend one arm straight out and hold for as long as is comfortable.

Then repeat on the other side.

ALTERNATE LEGS AND ARMS (kneeling superman)

As above, raising the opposite arm and leg.

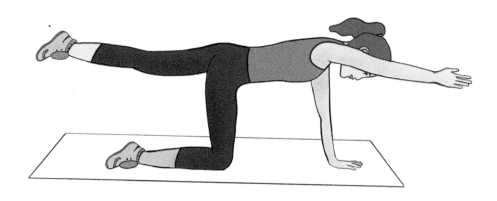

Alternate legs and arms (kneeling superman)

CRAWLING

This movement will strengthen all your spinal muscles.

On a mat, with leggings/trackies protecting your knees, crawl forward, then crawl back. Or crawl around a room at home.

ADVANCED CRAWL DOWNS

- Stand in front of the mat.

- Walk on your hands forward with your weight on them to get into a plank position from standing.

- To do this, slightly bend your knees and reach down to the floor with your hands for four counts until you are in a plank position (see page 66), then reverse the movement until you are upright again.

- Build up from one repetition to 10 x 3 sets.

BEGINNER ABDOMINAL EXERCISE LYING FACE DOWN (also great after pregnancy)

- Lie flat on your stomach.

- Your head should be resting on your hands with your face looking downwards and you should feel comfortable.

- You can also concentrate on your pelvic floor while doing this exercise. Focus on drawing in your pelvic floor muscles.

- Focus on keeping your ribs and hips on the floor.

- Now try to suck in your stomach. When strong, your abs should be slightly lifted off the floor so you can slide a hand under.

- Make sure you are lying straight as you can so your hips are evenly placed on the mat or floor. Your body should be totally relaxed.

- Breathing correctly is really important with this exercise. Breathe in through your nose as your abs are sucked in and lifted, hold for 10 seconds and then exhale through your mouth slowly as you relax your abs.

- Repeat this exercise up to 10 times.

This exercise may make you feel a bit nauseous, if you hold your breath, because of lack of oxygen so really concentrate on breathing at the same time as performing it; as soon as you stop performing it for a minute, the feeling will pass.

This exercise is a great starting point to build your abs back without straining your neck or spine.

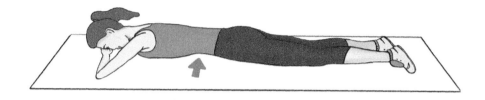

Beginner abdominal exercise lying face down
Head, hips, ribs on the floor; abs sucked in and lifted off the floor

PLANKING (using elbows)

This works the core and entire body.

To get into position, start on your hands and knees on a mat. Then lift your knees off the mat and push your feet back, extending your body and pressing your toes into the mat, making sure they are hip-width apart; keeping your hips elevated and not dipping them, bring your arms down so you are resting on your forearms at shoulder width. Do not let your shoulders dip.

Another way to get into a plank position is to kneel down, then rest on your forearms and extend your legs out, lifting your shoulders. Your elbows should be directly under your shoulders in a right-angle position.

Always have your hips lifted when planking. Do not listen to anyone who tells you to plank horizontal/level – doing so will put too much pressure on your back. Lifting your hips is far more effective as you will really feel your abs engage.

Concentrate on drawing in your lower abdominal muscles, pulling them inwards towards your spine.

Whether on your elbows or standing hand, the same technique applies.

To come down gently, bring your knees to the mat and sit gently back on your heels.

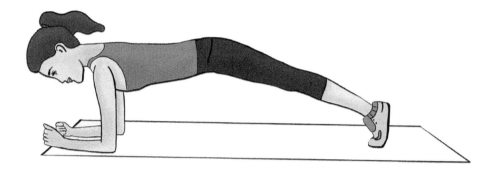

SIDE PLANKING

This works the core and the obliques.

Tip: look in the mirror to check your positioning.

Beginners side plank

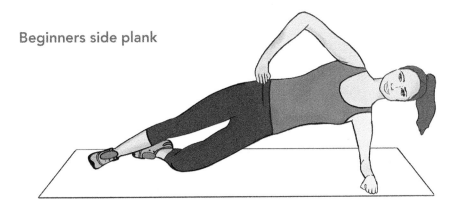

Side plank

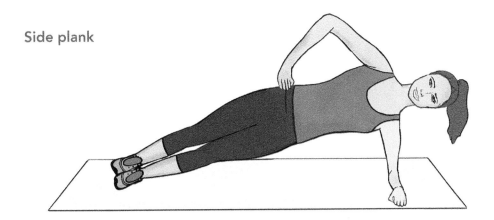

BEGINNER'S SIDE PLANK

- Lie on your side with your lower leg bent. Leave this leg on the floor. Your upper leg should be straight, stacked over the lower leg, resting the inside of the foot on the floor.

- Place your elbow directly under your shoulder.

- Lift your hips upwards so that the side of your body forms a straight line.

- Maintain a straight spinal alignment which means that your head and body and toes should follow each other in a straight line.

- Do not dip your hips.

- Do not let your hips or shoulders tilt forward or back.

- Keep your neck and head straight so that they are in line with your spine

- Start holding the position for 5 seconds, aiming for 60 seconds when you feel ready.

- Don't forget to breathe.

- Come down slowly and carefully to the floor.

- Repeat on the other side.

SIDE PLANK

This requires the same body position as the Beginner's Side Plank but stack your feet, one on top of the other, as shown on page 67.

Body balance

These exercises played a huge part in my recovery after my third surgery. I started with just holding a High Plank (see below) for a few seconds, then trying again a day or so later. This was from six weeks to six months, by which time I could do variations for the length of a full music track. They really power up your lats. They also work your core and biceps and stretch your hamstrings – a great all-over body workout. They will increase your strength and stamina.

Build up these sequences from just one to 20 repetitions as strength and stamina increase.

HIGH PLANK
(also known as 'top-of-push-up position')

A High Plank is similar to a typical elbow plank, as described on page 65, except your arms are extended in a push-up position, fully locked out. It decreases the leverage and is therefore easier to hold. It is used for Body Balance/planking variations.

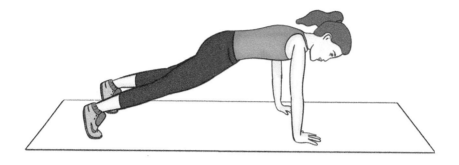

HIGH PLANK – EXERCISE VARIATIONS

Start on your hands and knees and with straight arms, shoulder-width apart. Lift your knees off the floor, pushing your toes into the floor. Please note that the direction in which to place the hands is different for most of my clients, depending on the individual alignment of their arms and what is comfortable for them.

Tip: If you find standing on your hands in this position a strain on your wrists you can use small push-up hand bars for support (under £10 easily found on a search online).

Your neck and head should continue along the same line as your spine so that your body is aligned. Lifting your head up will shorten your neck muscles; dropping your head will pull on your neck muscles, possibly resulting in neck strain and muscle pain, so ask your physiotherapist/personal trainer and/or check in the mirror you are in the correct position.

Make sure your pelvis and hips are elevated slightly (so not in a total straight line) to take the pressure off your lower spine. Do not dip your hips, nor arch your back. Do draw (suck) in your abs (stomach muscles).

From the High Plank position a number of combination Body Balance exercises can be performed. These exercises will strengthen your lats (back muscles) and your abs.

HIGH PLANK AND DOWNWARD-FACING DOG

This elongates and releases tension from the spine and opens out the hips and shoulders. It also stretches the hamstrings and calves and strengthens the entire body, especially the abs and lats.

The starting position is the High Plank.

Draw your abs (stomach muscles) in towards your navel.

Make sure you do not scrunch up your shoulders around your neck. Keep them drawn down towards your tailbone. This will also help you to engage your lats and use them correctly.

You can keep your knees straight (or bend them a little if your hamstrings - backs of your legs - are very tight). You do not have to have your heels on the ground. You can lift them or be on the balls of your feet and tip toes. Play around with this to see which you prefer.

Draw your lower rib area and abs inwards as you lift your pelvis, hips and tailbone upwards into a downward-facing dog pose (see illustration). Push your chest downwards, towards the floor. In the mirror you should be making an upside down 'V' shape with your body. Imagine someone is pulling your hips towards the ceiling.

Hold this pose for a few seconds and then bring your body back to the starting position of the High Plank. Again, be careful not to arch your

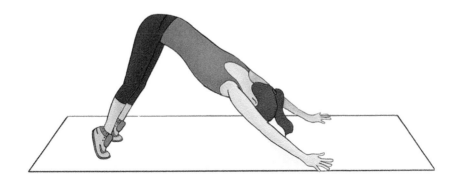

back or dip your pelvis and hips.

Hold the pose for a few seconds and then repeat. Start with two repetitions and then build up to eight. You can increase over time adding extra sets and extra repetitions.

Once you are really strong you can try these more advanced combinations:

– High Plank and Downward-facing Dog with Mini Press-up

– High Plank with Bear Squats

– High Plank with Mountain Climbers

HIGH PLANK AND DOWNWARD-FACING DOG ADDING A MINI PRESS-UP

This is exactly the same as the High Plank and Downward Facing Dog combination but when you return back to the High Plank try adding one mini press-up. The order of the exercise should be like this:

High Plank to

Downward Facing Dog to

High Plank to

Mini Press-Up

returning to the High Plank position

Then repeat up to 10 times.

HIGH PLANK AND BEAR SQUATS

This combination works your quad and glute muscles, as well as your lats and abs and arms.

Get yourself into the High Plank position.

Bear squat

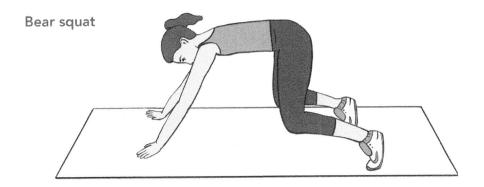

Now, instead of keeping your knees straight, bend them and sit/squat horizontally, bringing your glutes/bottom back, and gently stretching your arms. Keep your abs drawn in towards your navel, your back straight and your head in line with your body. Again, do not look down or upwards.

Hold for a few seconds.

Perform this exercise slowly and with control.

Then return to the High Plank position.

Build up from one to 10 repetitions.

The Bear Squat is often performed pushing the glutes/bottom towards the ceiling and straightening the legs. However, I feel that this will put a strain on the lower back and also the shoulders, which is not advisable for scoliosis/spinal-fusion patients.

HIGH PLANK WITH MOUNTAIN CLIMBERS (advanced)

This is an exercise to speed up your heart rate while firing up nearly every muscle group in your body and increasing your general strength.

It works the deltoids, biceps, triceps, chest muscles, abs, obliques, quads, hamstrings and hip abductors.

The starting position is the High Plank.

With your feet hip-width apart, bring your right knee towards your chest, pulling your abs in tight so that you do not sag/dip your hips down, and making sure you retain your High Plank position.

Take your right leg back and swap legs.

You should begin this exercise slowly and with control. Once you have mastered the technique you can speed up a little.

Be careful to be very soft on your feet. Do not bang them down as a heavy impact will reverberate through your spine.

Start with a maximum of six repetitions and build up to three sets of 20 repetitions over time.

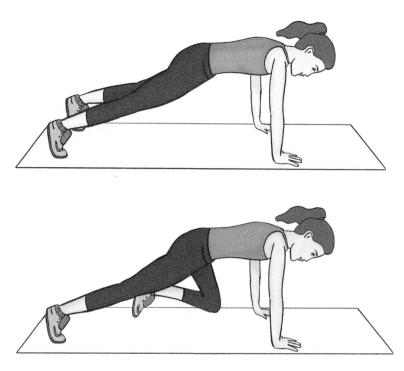

Gym equipment

There is a large selection of machines to use in most gyms. Many of these work the same muscle groups. If you are training without a physiotherapist or personal trainer, do make sure you are familiar with the machines. Check that the machine you plan to use suits the particular alignment of your back, so you are comfortable performing the exercise.

General rule: if it hurts, STOP.

Do not be tempted to overload and increase the amount you lift so that you are unable to perform 20 repetitions easily.

Start at 5 kg.

Depending on the machine, do not go above 10 kg.

Start with six repetitions. If this is challenging, reduce the weight.

Increase repetitions and sets slowly.

Lat pulldown machine

This is one of my favourites. It works your lats and it is great as a starting point once the okay has been given to exercise.

Before you attempt to use this machine, adjust the level of the seating position. You should be able to sit down with your knees under the rests. If on a ball, it should be firm.

Your feet should be 1½ hip-width apart. Your knees should follow the alignment of your toes. Make sure your knees are not over your toes.

The position you work out in and sit in on a day-to-day basis is super important. Sitting with your toes under your knees will put pressure on your knees. You have enough issues with your back – you really don't want knee problems too.

The trainer or physio will pull the bar down. If training alone, reach for the bar with arms 1½ shoulder-distance apart using an overhand grip.

- Correct your sitting knee alignment position.
- Suck your abs in.
- Sit upright leaning 2 cm back (that's hardly at an angle).
- Pull the bar down to your upper chest and then release it gently so that your elbows do not bounce or hyperextend.
- Start with no weight and just the bar with five repetitions.

THEN SLIGHTLY CHANGE THE EXERCISE:

- Have your arms narrow with underhand grip.
- Double check that your hips, knees and toes are in alignment and that your toes are slightly turned out to 11:00 pm and 1:00 pm. Your knees should not be over your toes. The angle of your bent knees – the distance between the back of your thighs and your

calves – should not exceed 90 degrees to avoid strain on your knees.

- Suck in your abs.

- Sit upright leaning a little further back (4 cm). Looking upwards, pull the bar down to your upper chest and then release gently so that your elbows do not bounce or hyperextend.

- Start with no weight and just the bar with five repetitions.

If it is the first time you are training after surgery, just take your time, adding just one or two extra repetitions each time you train. Once you can do 20 repetitions x 3 sets, it is time to add the 5-kg weight on the machine.

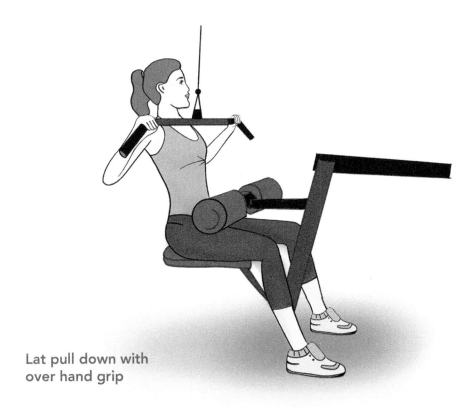

Lat pull down with over hand grip

Assisted dip machine

This is excellent for toning your lats and tri's safely.

This machine looks a bit scary in the gym, but once you've been shown how to use it, the progression of recovery and getting strength back can be amazing.

It looks confusing as the weight level is in reverse.

Take your body weight, e.g. 62 kg, and put the weight level at 60 kg – you are then lifting 2 kg of your body weight. As the weight is reduced, the intensity of the exercise increases.

Kneel on the knee rest. Suck in your abs and tilt your pelvis slightly. Do not hyperextend your arms.

This machine can also be used for Assisted Lat Pulldowns, using the same body position as the dips but reaching up to place your hands on the high bar. See pages 76, 77 for instructions.

There are two variations:

1. Wide-arm pulls with an overhand grip.

2. Shoulder-width arm pulls with underhand grip, leaning slightly back.

Start with low repetitions (five) and increase with progression.

Assisted dip machine performing an Assisted Tricep Dip

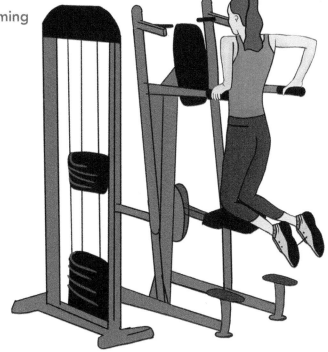

- Step onto machine and then kneel carefully on the pad and at the same time place your hands on the dip bars and bend your elbows, keeping your back straight.

- Slowly lower your body down until your arms make a 90 degree angle.

- Push yourself back to your starting position without hyperextending your arms or locking them out. Be soft on your elbows.

- Repeat five times to start with, building to 10, and then start to add a second set.

- Be mindful of your footing when you get down from the machine. You cannot twist your back to get off, so if you feel you may need help, make sure someone is around to guide you before you start.

Seated row

This is really good for building all back muscles - that is, lats, rhomboid, erector spinae.

- Adjust the seat as for the lat pulldown machine.

- Hold your core in. Sit upright. If the machine has a chest rest, sit at 90°.

SEATED CABLE ROW EXERCISE STEPS

Starting position

Sit upright on the bench, facing the low-pulley row machine. (Some seated row machines have a bar, often described as a 'V-bar' as it is V-shaped, some have two separate handles on cables.)

Keep your feet up on the front platform, making sure your knees are slightly bent.

Lean over, keeping the natural alignment of your back, and grab the bar.

Keep your arms extended and pull back your torso so that it makes a right angle with your legs – then lean just 2 cm back.

Suck in your core so that your torso is static, shoulders down, relaxed.

Next

- Keeping your torso stationary, pull the handles of the bar back towards you. Breathe out, keep your arms close to your body, and pull the bar until your thumbs touch your abs. Squeeze your back muscles.

- Do not lean forward or back after pulling the bar. Avoid moving your body. It is just your arms moving and your chest is pushed out as your back muscles are squeezed together.

- Hold this pose for a second.
- Slowly release the contraction and go back to the starting position.
- As your arms extend, make sure you control the cable, releasing it slowly to avoid your elbows bouncing, your arms hyperextending and your body jolting forwards.
- Do not initiate the pull with your shoulder muscles – use your lats.
- Start with 6 reps. Build to 20 x 3 over time.

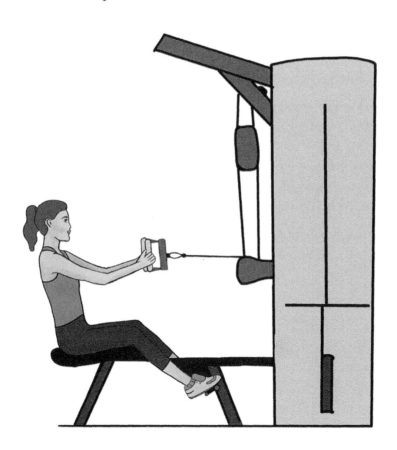

Free weights

Do not go above a total of 5 kg. It is not necessary. You will still get great results. In my opinion, it should take from 6 months to 2½ years after surgery to build up to 5 kg, with a maximum of three sets of 20-30 repetitions for each exercise, depending on the exercise.

Start all free-weight exercises by just making a fist without using a weight. Get your body used to the movements. After surgery, muscles may have been cut and/or not used for a while. Even just a few repetitions without a weight may cause muscle fatigue. Introduce each exercise very slowly. Wait a couple of days to check how the muscle has reacted to each exercise. Then progress.

Training sensibly, starting with a few minutes and building up to an hour over time, will give you toned muscles. Your body can look amazing.

Lunges (static)

Lunges are great for building up quads and glutes.

Always have your feet hip-width apart for balance. Focus on your hips being square on.

Think right-angles. Your knees and ankles should be no lower than 90° – your knees should not peep over your toes. Take a step forward and tippy toe on your back foot. Focus on static lunges to start with, by building your lunge position with one foot forward and the other foot back, moving your body up and down. Do not bang your knees on the floor.

Six repetitions building up to 20 x 5 sets on each leg.

Start without weights and build up to a maximum of 2 kg in each hand over a year or so.

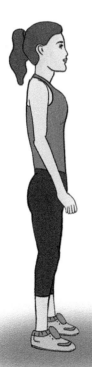
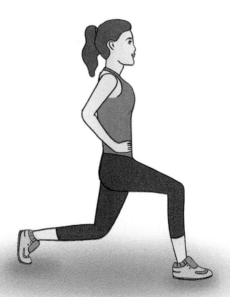

MOVING LUNGES

Use alternate legs, keeping your legs hip-width apart, hips square on, retaining your balance.

Step your right foot forward, lunge downwards and then bring your right leg back to the starting position.

Repeat on the other side.

Pay attention to your posture: upright, facing forwards.

Build up as for static lunges.

WALKING LUNGES

Do these on your walks from six months after surgery.

They are great for building stamina and strength and giving legs great shape. I often walk the streets doing these! Neighbours can only make so many jokes about how I/my clients look and now they are bored. So ignore odd looks.

These are the same as moving lunges except carry on lunging with alternate legs. Alternate walking and lunging.

Squats

The configuration of a fused spine means that squats must be adapted. Your body may be more forward than most other people's performing these. That is okay. You need to hold your abs very tight.

Make sure your knees do not go over your toes – stick your bottom out and go as if to sit down without touching the seat. And never let your bottom go lower than your knees.

Do not overload on weight. Start without any weights. Only introduce a light weight after at least nine months.

Squats can incorporate upright rowing (page 90) to increase stamina.

Normal (hip width), wide-leg and ski squats (legs together) are all safe.

Start with 10 squats and increase level as you feel stronger up to 30 x 3–5 sets.

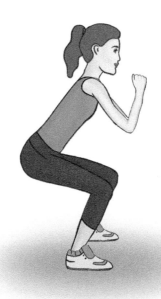

Bent-arm pullovers

This is my favourite exercise of all time! This is because it works your lats, and your rhoms, rear delts, pecs and tri's (back, rear shoulder muscle, chest and the lower back muscle on your arm from armpit to above the elbow) all in one go – all the while, supporting your back, neck and head, so it's very safe and effective in my opinion. When adding a weight, scoliosis patients working out alone need to ask someone trained to help.

You will often see people do this exercise on a bench. Use a mat instead, as it is easier to get up after by rolling on your side.

1. Lie on your back.

2. Position your feet a little wider apart than hip width, hips following the alignment of your knees, ankles and toes.

3. Head position: look upwards, with your head resting on the mat, your chin tucked in but relaxed.

4. Press back into the floor with your pelvis tilted upwards. You can use a wedge to help with this position if you like.

5. Start by just clasping your hands together into a fist. Progress by adding weights up to max 5 kg.

6. Have your elbows slightly bent. Start with your arms at eyeline, held over your chest, then extend them above your head. Due to scoliosis, your shoulders will find their own comfortable position. Do not force your shoulders. Only extend your arms as far as is comfortable. A slight stretch will be felt.

7. Keep your back into the mat by sucking in your abs.

8. Breathe out through your mouth on the way up and in through your nose on the way down.

9. It is only your shoulder joints that are moving. Just move your slightly bent arms from directly above your chest, bringing the arms to your ear level and then back again to eye level above the chest. Do not attempt to bring your arms further back to touch the floor behind you as this will make you arch your back.

10. Start with five repetitions with no weight and increase to 5 kg and 20 repetitions x 3 sets.

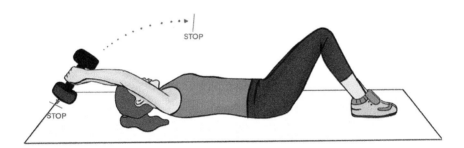

Lying-down flys

This exercise works the pecs (chest), deltoids (shoulders) and biceps muscles.

Use the same positioning as for the bent-arm pullover (page 86).

Start with just your fists, not the weights shown opposite. Your muscles will be very weak after surgery; remember, some may have been cut.

Looking upwards, make your fists meet above your chest, bend your elbows slightly and extend your arms outwards, leading with your elbows. Make sure your wrists and arms are fixed – it is only the shoulder joint that should be used. Do not land with your elbows or arms on the floor. Start with a small movement.

As strength increases, add small weights, but not to more than 3 kg on each side. When adding weights your physio or trainer should be spotting for (helping) you.

Start with three repetitions and build to 20 repetitions x 3 sets.

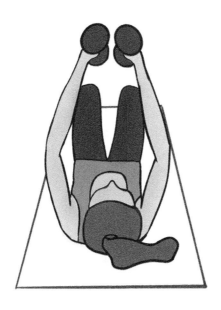

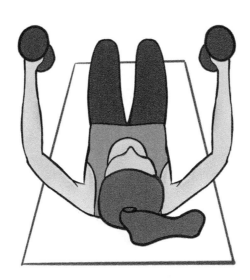

Upright row

The upright row works the traps – the triangular muscle at top of the spine that connects to the deltoids.

I am a huge fan of this exercise. It is so important to keep the trapezius muscle toned. It helps to hold your head upright. If you look around you will see some elderly people who walk with their head hung forward – this may be partly due to very weak traps. This exercise will also tone the flabby bit some people have at the back of their neck. If performed regularly, it can take up to six months to tone this area and really feel the benefits. Just start with six repetitions and build up to 15 and increase up to three sets. If you feel neck and shoulder strain after this exercise, just reduce the repetitions next time.

This exercise really does work and in my opinion is essential. Clients have reported to me that in the long term it has improved their posture and in turn reduced neck aches and headaches.

- Stand with your legs hip-width apart.

- Your knees should be soft and slightly bent, and your shoulders relaxed.

- Start with your arms down at thigh level, relaxed holding the bar with your hands thumb-width apart. Leading with your elbows, slowly raise the bar, your hands brushing your body until they are at upper chest level and your elbows are higher than your hands and are elevated above your shoulders, making the shape of a V (see diagram opposite).

- Do not be tempted to raise your shoulders; keep them down.

- Slowly return to the starting position.

- Introduce a weighted bar or free weights really slowly, starting with 0.5 kg, to a maximum of 3 kg.

Upright row

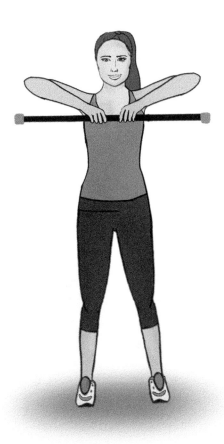

Side-to-side obliques

- These work the side abs.

- Stand with your knees slightly bent, legs hip-width apart.

- Suck in your core. Have your pelvis slightly tilted and your shoulders relaxed.

- Start with a slight movement, bending your waist to one side, return to standing, then bend to the other side.

- Take care not to push your hips out to the side – they should be square on. Do not swing.

- Start with just a few repetitions without weights.

- Progress by increasing the number of repetitions to a maximum of 20 x 3 sets and maximum of 2 kg free weights.

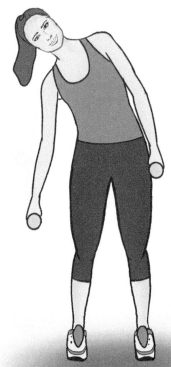

Standing beginner abs with free weights
(a John Rutherford exercise)

This exercise works the core:

- Stand with your feet hip-width apart, your pelvis slightly tilted forward and your shoulders relaxed
  OR

- sit on a chair with your feet out in front of you, making sure your knees are not over your toes

- Check that the alignment of your hips, knees, ankles and toes follow through in the same direction.

- Make a fist with both hands.

- Imagine you are walking fast and your arms are swinging with your elbows bent. Hold your core tight, only your arms should be moving, with your elbows bent. Move your arms as quickly as you can, while holding your core still.

- To build up intensity add light free weights up to 2 kg.

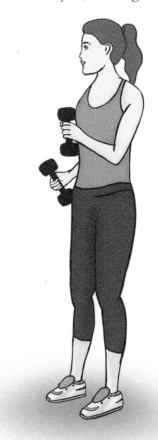

Free-weight deltoid raises

- This exercise works the shoulder muscles.

- Use weights from 0.5 kg to a max of 3 kg.

- Stand or sit upright on a chair, feet in front of toes, suck in your core and make sure your shoulders are relaxed down. Do not be tempted to bring your shoulders up to your ears when you raise your elbows. Start without weights, just using your fists.

- Bend your elbows to no more than 90°.

- Leading with your elbows and keeping your wrists strong, raise your elbows outwards to less than 90°. Do not raise them higher than your shoulders – that would put too much stress on the side neck muscles after surgery.

- Come back to the starting position.

- Only repeat a few times: I would recommend a maximum of six to eight repetitions and a limit of two sets at any time.

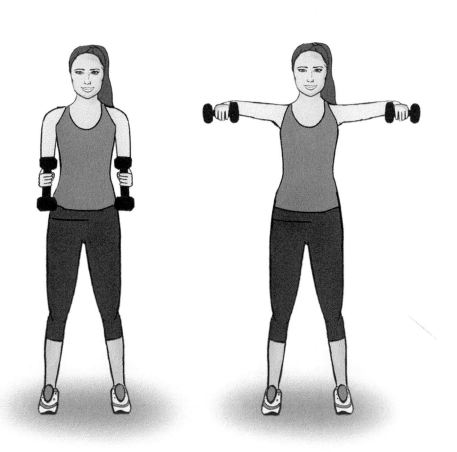

TRX training
Suspension training

The TRX System was developed by a Navy Seal so he could train to stay in shape in small spaces using minimal equipment. It leverages gravity and body weight to build strength, endurance and balance, while it activates your core (back, chest, abs) and works your arms and legs too. It is suitable for all levels of training and I used it as part of my steps to recovery from surgery two years ago.

For trainers and physios – you know what you are doing.

For home purchasing, TRX has to be secure - see product information and take advice from the TRX Suspension Training website on fixings on their website trxtraining.co.uk.

If you are a scoliosis patient, it is worth paying for at least one or two sessions with a trainer or physio to show you how to use the TRX.

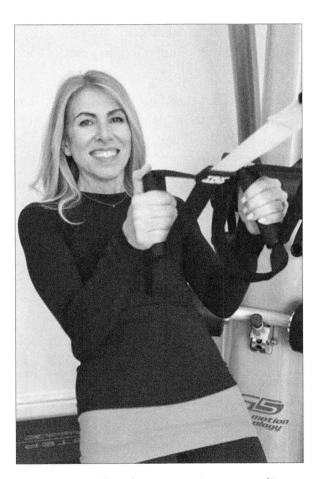

TRX standing low row – in my studio

The standing low row

This exercise works all the muscles in the back.

It is excellent for posture issues.

The straps should be short to start with. Increase the difficulty over time by lengthening the straps and walking your feet in so you are at more of an angle.

- Stand facing the anchor point holding on to the handles, then lean back with your arms straight, with palms facing each other.

- Pull your body towards the anchor point and squeeze your shoulder blades.

- Return to the start.

- Start with six repetitions and build up to 20, adding up to three sets. As the exercise becomes easier, increase the difficulty level by lengthening the straps and walking your feet further forward, as I have said. Make sure your trainers have a good grip so that there is no danger of you slipping forward.

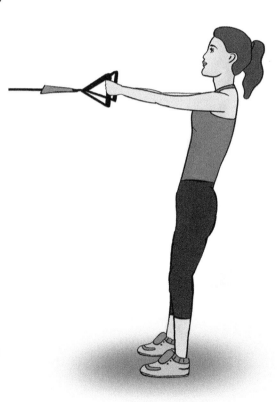

THE TRX PIKE

This exercise works the core, abs, lats and hip flexors. It is a very advanced exercise for those who have built up their strength and stability to a high level. The definition of a 'pike' is bending your body in half at the hips so your hips are elevated and your legs are straight.

After two years of training/recovery and if you/your client have/has the strength and stamina, there is no reason not to perform a pike on the TRX. Look at the spine of the woman in the picture on the next page (page 100) – it is straight.

- Start kneeling away from the anchor point with both feet in the cradles and your hands under your shoulders.

- Lift your knees so you are in a plank position with your hips slightly lifted.

- Raise your hips up, sucking in your abs and pelvic floor.

- Keep your legs straight.

- Lower your body back to the starting position.

- Do this exercise very slowly, starting with three repetitions only. Build up to 15 repetitions x 3 sets when you are very strong.

If you are reading this chapter and you are pre-surgery, obviously you will have more flexibility and will not be as restricted as some.

Physiotherapists will have their own exercises and stretches to give you which should be followed and, again, check my stretches on pages 110-118 will work for you within your spinal fusion limitations.

High Plank

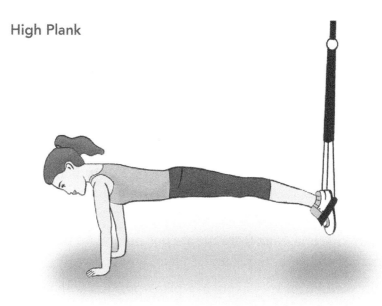

The TRX Pike

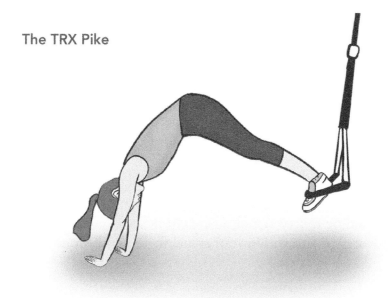

Other useful approaches

SWISS BALL/EXERCISE BALLS
(also see page 48)

Caution! Balls are great for sitting on or using to elevate your legs when lying on your back to take the pressure off your lower spine. I would caution against raising hips or using a ball as a bench to do free weights, in case you lose balance, fall over and twist.

YOGA

Yoga is lovely for stretching. Some moves will be very limiting, but please don't let that put you off. Go to a good teacher who understands scoliosis. Adelene Cheong at TRIYOGA in Camden Town, London, is excellent and runs yoga workshops for people with scoliosis. Performed correctly, taking into account your anatomy, after a yoga session you should feel incredible.

PILATES RING

This is a really useful piece of equipment.

Use it for inside-thigh adductor strengthening.

This exercise will tone your inner thighs quite quickly as the adductor muscle is small and generally reacts well to isolated toning exercise.

- Lie on the floor, feet hip-width apart, back pressed gently into the floor, pelvis slightly tilted, head and shoulders relaxed. Feel free to add a wedge for support under your hips.

- Place the Pilates ring between your thighs, just above your knees, as shown below, and squeeze your thighs together.

- Start with 10 repetitions and build up to 100 very slowly to avoid groin strain.

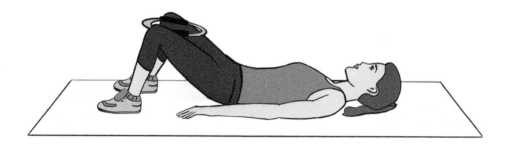

Inside-thigh adductor exercise using a Pilates ring with the pelvis slightly tilted.

Resistance exercise bands

Resistence exercise bands are a great alternative to weights and easy to start using on your own, with you deciding your own tension. They are easy to store too.

Resistence bands come in several strengths and are generally labelled as follows, depending on the manufacturer:

Light (yellow)

Medium (red)

Heavy (green)

Extra strong (blue)

Adjust where you hold the band to achieve the right amount of flexibility for you.

I would recommend these for stretching too, as described in the next section. Unfortunately, I cannot put every exercise into this guide; some tried-and-tested safe suggestions follow on pages 104-109.

LYING-DOWN ABDUCTOR EXTENSION WITH BAND AROUND THIGHS

This exercise works the outer thighs

- Lie on your back with your knees bent and pelvis tilted upwards, your back pushed into the floor and your upper body relaxed. You can have an optional wedge under your bottom/upper thigh area.

- Place your feet wide apart and a strong band above your knees, as shown.

- Push your legs outwards then bring legs back to start position, keeping the band taut.

- Start with 20 repetitions x 1, building to 30 x 3 sets. You can also try little pulses keeping the band taut.

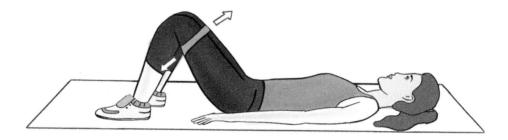

SIDE-STEPS: ABDUCTORS AND HIP FLEXOR

- Put a good music track on.

- Standing position.

- Place the band around either your ankles, lower legs or upper thighs – whichever is most comfortable for you – but not around your knees.

- The band should have tension, no slack; your knees should be slightly bent and chest up. Your stance should be outside of hip width.

- Slowly side step, keeping the band tight for 10 repetitions to one side and then repeat back to your starting position.

- Build repeats until you can manage the length of the music track.

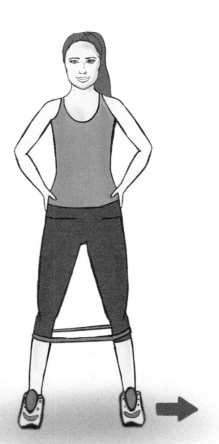

ARMS ABOVE HEAD

This exercise works the lats, traps, rhoms, bi's and core:

- Stand with your feet 1½ hip-width apart, your core static and held in, and your knees slightly bent.

- Hold the band in both hands.

- Extend your arms above your head with your elbows slightly bent outwards and your wrists straight.

- Keep the band taut.

- Pull out slowly for 10 seconds, hold for 10, pulse for 10. Repeat.

- Build up from one set to three.

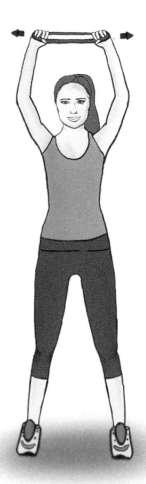

ARMS BEHIND BACK
(a John Rutherford exercise)

This exercise works the rhoms, tri's and core.

- Use a really easy band to try this.

- Posture: core held in, feet hip-width apart, checking your hip alignment follows through to your knees and in turn follows your ankles to toes, with knees slightly bent and shoulders relaxed.

- With your arms behind your back, band in your hands, wrists straight and strong have your elbows slightly bent outwards.

- Pull your hands away from each other for 10 repetitions, keeping tension of the band. Relax.

- Repeat, building up to 3 sets.

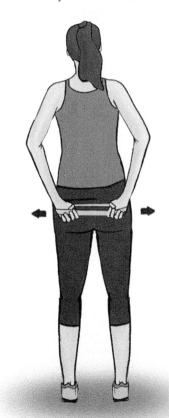

CHEST FLYS WITH BAND

This exercise works the pecs – the chest muscles – without overloading the shoulders.

- Lie down on your back, with your back gently pushed into the mat, pelvis tilted upwards, knees bent 1½ hip-widths apart, following alignment to your toes.

- Have your arms above your chest, elbows slightly bent and wrists fixed.

- Hold the band in your fists and pull open, keeping the tension at all times.

- Pull slowly, hold for a count of 10, then release, still retaining the tension on the band. Perform 10 repetitions, adding another set when you feel stronger and/or increase the resistance of the band.

- Build up to 3 sets.

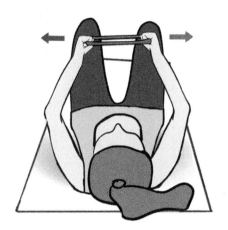

SEATED ROW BAND

This exercise works the lats – the back muscles.

- Sit on the mat, legs in front and knees bent, pelvis tilted upwards.

- Suck your abs in, leaning slightly back. Keep the shoulders relaxed.

- With the band looped around you feet, pull it towards your chest, sticking your chest out but keeping your back static, then relax your arms forwards gently, without hyperextending your elbows. Do not arch your back or move forward and back as if rowing a boat.

- Breathe out through your mouth as you pull on the band towards your body and breathe in as you relax the tension on the band bringing it forward.

- Start with six repetitions. Build up to 20 x 3 sets.

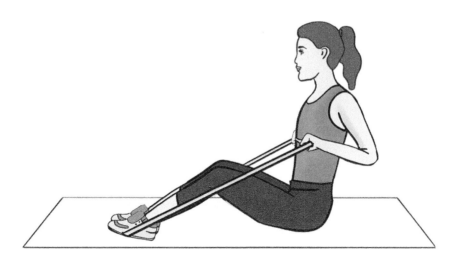

Stretching

Physiotherapists will have their own stretches to give you, which should be followed. Please check that the following stretches will work for you within your spinal fusion limitations.

If you are reading this chapter and have not had scoliosis surgery, you will obviously have more flexibility and will not be as restricted.

Be very gentle with your body when you stretch. If you do not feel comfortable at any time, STOP.

Stretches are for the end of your workout or once you are warm, e.g. after a good walk. It is not advisable to stretch cold muscles as you may tear/pull a muscle.

It is not necessary to stretch so deeply that your muscles start to shake.

Do not bounce/pulse your stretch as there is a danger of pinging/pulling a muscle.

The key to stretching is to feel tension in the muscle you are stretching.

Once the tension relaxes, you can then try to slowly go into a deeper stretch.

BANISTER STRETCH

This is my all-time favourite stretch. It is my go-to stretch for any client who walks into my studio complaining that they have 'done something' to their back, or when I just want a lovely waking-up stretch. If you sit at a desk for work, the banister stretch is great for pulling out a compressed spine, opening up your vertebrae.

- Find a banister or fixed pole.

- Feet one and a half hip width apart

- Grip with your hands and squat down and outwards.

- Keep your back flat, head in line with your body, core sucked in.

- Do not arch your back.

- Imagine someone is pulling your hips towards the back of the room. Sit further down to get a deeper spinal stretch.

- Hold for a few seconds up to 60, and repeat.

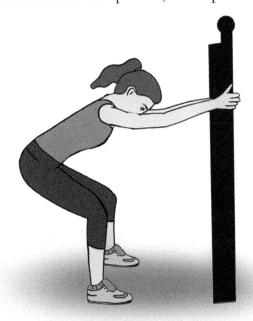

ALTERNATE CHILD'S POSE

- Start on all fours.

- Feet together, knees far apart.

- Keep you back flat, and your head in line with your body.

- Sit back just above your heels.

- Push your chest towards the ground without arching your back.

- Arms in front, fingers outstretched.

- Take a breath in through your nose and hold it for five seconds. As you breathe out through your mouth, crawl your fingers further forward to get a really lovely back stretch.

- Repeat a few times.

- To get up, suck your abs and rib cage in tightly, making sure that you do not arch your back, to bring you back to the start position on all fours.

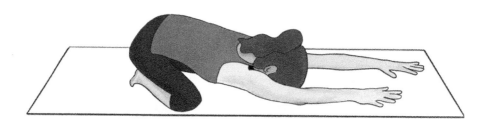

HAND HANGING

I find this stretch a great relief.

- Find a high bar or top of a door you can just reach.

- Hold with both hands. Bend your knees and try to sit, so you are dropping your spine downwards. Do not arch your back, but suck your abs in.

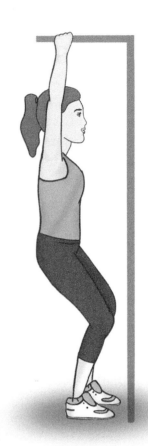

LOWER-BACK MASSAGE STRETCH

- Lie on your back.

- Hug your knees into your stomach.

- Gently circle your legs together in one direction x 3 circles.

- Hug your knees in, then repeat circling them in the other direction.

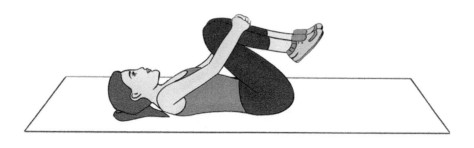

If your legs feel tight

HAMSTRING STRETCH WITH BAND

Lie flat on your back with one knee bent. You will often see instructors/people doing this stretch with the lower leg straight. This is not advisable for scoliosis patients due to the configuration of your spine – leaving a leg bent with one foot on the floor will keep the pressure off.

Leave your head on the floor; do not be tempted to raise it as you have a good chance of giving yourself neck ache and will put pressure on the cervical (neck) and upper thoracic (upper back) area.

Decide which strength of band to use (see page 103).

- Wrap the band around your foot and gently pull the foot upwards.

- Do not bounce it.

- Try to straighten the raised leg.

- Hold for 5-30 seconds.

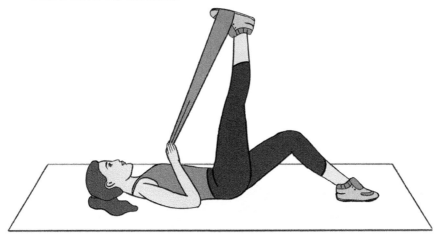

Hamstring stretch and starting position for Lying down hip stretch and Groin stretch/inner thigh stretch

LYING HIP STRETCH

- Position is the same as for the Hamstring Stretch (page 114).

- Using your left hand to pull the band which is looped around your left foot with your left leg raised, take this leg gently across your body to your right holding on tightly to the band.

- Do not force the stretch and take your leg too far across as you do not want to twist your lower back.

- You should feel this stretch in your glutes (bottom).

- Hold for 5 to 20 seconds.

- Move back to the starting position.

- Repeat on the other side.

GROIN STRETCH/INNER THIGH STRETCH

- Position is the same as for the Hamstring Stretch (page 114).

- Using your left hand to pull the band which is looped around your left foot with your left leg raised, take this leg gently outwards holding on tightly to the band to avoid straining your inside thigh (adductor muscles).

- Increase the stretch slowly.

- Hold for 5 to 20 seconds.

- Move the leg back to the starting position.

- Repeat on the other side.

GLUTE AND HIP STRETCH

- Position is the same as for the Hamstring Stretch.

- With your left leg raised, loop the band round your left foot and grab the band with one or both hands.

- Bend the knee of your raised left leg outwards and place your left foot over the opposite bent right leg just above the knee. Gently pull your left foot towards you with the band that is wrapped around it.

- You can choose to slowly raise your right foot off the ground to feel a deeper stretch.

- Hold for 5 to 20 seconds

- Repeat on the other side.

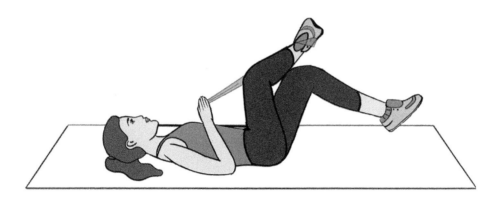

Glute and hip stretch (with foot raised off the ground for a deeper stretch)

SEATED OBLIQUE STRETCH
(a John Rutherford exercise)

This movement offers excellent release.

- Sit on a chair, bench or Swiss ball (see pages 48 and 101 for guidance) with your knees at a 90° angle.

- Cross your arms above your head with your hands on opposite shoulders.

- Really try to sit up as tall as you can.

- Move gently from one side to the other, lifting your hips off the chair alternately.

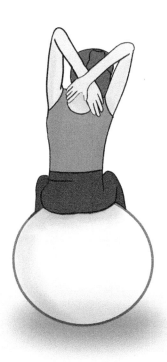

STANDING NECK PUSH AGAINST WALL
(a John Rutherford exercise)

This movement could come under exercises OR stretching depending on how slowly it is done. I recommend super slow.

It works the neck muscles and helps with strengthening the neck and improving posture.

- Stand with your back to the wall and your knees slightly bent.

- Gently push your head back using your neck muscles to try to touch the wall at eye level.

- Make the push a very small movement towards the wall making sure your chin is tucked slightly in, hold for a few seconds, then relax.

- Repeat the pushes six times and build to 10 repetitions x 3 sets.

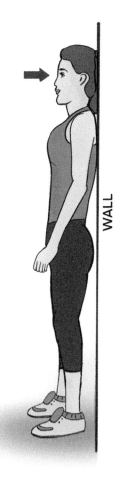

WALL

PREGNANCY AND SCOLIOSIS

§

Pregnancy and scoliosis

Please be guided by your doctor.

There is no reason why women should not have a healthy pregnancy and baby after scoliosis surgery.

I was advised to get super-fit in order to carry a baby and avoid having too much strain and pain. I can only go from my own experiences and share them.

Mr Tim Morley, who was my consultant at the time, told me that it is really important for the body to be as strong as possible before even considering having a baby post scoliosis surgery. I was at athletic peak fitness and strength when I gave birth to my children. Mr Morley's advice paid off. I experienced zero back pain throughout each pregnancy, even though I was vomiting violently every day with my second.

My physio at the time encouraged me to train really hard as I had been in a great deal of pain before my first pregnancy when I initially saw her. She said if I could get my stomach muscles strong, as well as my spinal muscles, I would be fine. She was a strong believer in short abdominal crunches – lots of them! Her theory was that the more developed the abdominals, the more support there would be for the baby. The baby would be carried high as the muscles would act as a strong support.

I trained so intensely that I had a visible six-pack. On one hospital visit, while I was being monitored, I was told by a very experienced, old-fashioned matron that she had never seen muscles so noticeable over a bump and freaked me out by saying that they would never go 'back to flat'. Thankfully she was completely wrong and my stomach was 'back to flat' relatively quickly.

Causes of back pain in pregnancy

Women without scoliosis can experience back pain during pregnancy. Pain typically occurs where the pelvis meets the spine, at the sacroiliac joint.

There are many possible reasons for pain. Here are some of the more likely:

WEIGHT GAIN

During a healthy pregnancy, women can typically gain between 11 and 16 kg. The spine has to support that weight and this can cause lower back pain. The weight of the growing baby and uterus also puts pressure on the blood vessels and nerves in the pelvis and back.

POSTURE CHANGES

Pregnancy shifts the centre of body gravity. As a result, pregnant women may gradually – even without noticing it – begin to adjust their posture and the way they move. This may result in back pain or strain. A fused spine could mean extra discomfort.

Everything becomes soft around the spine when pregnant and there is a school of thought that says the spine can move up to 7° during pregnancy. Having said that, as the years have passed and the explanations for spinal curvature have varied it is really hard to put a 'one-size-fits-all' label on it.

HORMONAL CHANGES

During pregnancy, the body creates a hormone called relaxin. This allows ligaments in the pelvic area to relax and the joints to become looser in preparation for the birth process. The same hormone can

121

cause ligaments that support the spine to loosen, leading to instability and pain.

MUSCLE SEPARATION

As the uterus expands, two parallel sheets of muscle (the rectus abdominis muscles), which run from the rib cage to the pubic bone, may separate along the centre seam. This separation may make back pain worse.

STRESS

Emotional stress can cause muscle tension in the back, which may be felt as back pain or back spasms. You may find that you experience an increase in back pain during stressful periods of your pregnancy.

Exercise in pregnancy

So which exercises can you do while pregnant? And which should you avoid?

The exercises in this guide should all be suitable to perform while pregnant, as long as they feel comfortable. (Always take professional advice.)

I'm not a huge fan of running long distances if you have back or knee problems, so it's obvious that I would advise you to steer clear of running while pregnant.

- Avoid any activity which entails jumping up and down/high impact.

- Lying on your stomach may not be comfortable or advisable.

- Reduce the amount of free weights and machine weight. Try using exercise bands as an alternative.

- The cross-trainer, rower and walking machines are all good in pregnancy. Walking is great.

'Well, I think that it's vital that women with scoliosis realise that pregnancy is not contraindicated and what's needed is a careful, joint approach with all the specialists involved and a mum who is really motivated to keep her body in the best possible shape.'

Peter Mason FRCS FRCOG
Consultant obstetrician and gynaecologist

Bathing a baby/toddler

I recommend getting someone else to help!

In scoliosis post surgery, the spine is fused, so kneeling over a bath, bathing and picking up a baby will cause strain in the upper thoracic spine. The vertebrae that are not fused will take the strain and this may cause soreness and discomfort.

If possible, arrange for a relative/friend/nanny/maternity nurse to come in for a couple hours to help, especially from newborn as this is when your back will be most vulnerable. Maternity nurses can be very expensive, so it is worth asking any newly qualified baby nurses/midwives if they can do a few nights at a more reasonable cost in order to gain some work experience. Ask in your ward at the hospital. Some agencies send their newly qualified maternity nurses out on work experience, so it's worth calling to ask.

Raising the baby bath on to the top of a surface at waist level will avoid stooping over.

TIPS
A-Z

AIRLINE TRAVEL

Take two neck cushions for support - one for your neck and the other for your back (also good for long train/coach journeys). The pillows provided by the airlines are usually useless. Take a soft blanket to wrap yourself in and a soft scarf for your neck. A cosy hoodie is also great for neck support if you scrunch up the hood into the back of your neck. Wear comfortable clothes. If you are stuck in a window seat and desperate, kick your shoes off and try to elevate your legs, bending your knees, resting them on the back of the armrest in front of you. I know this is not ideal advice but it's better than being in agony.

Try to book an aisle seat or a seat at the front/extra legroom, so you have more space to stretch your legs out.

For any flight over three hours or long haul make sure you get up and walk around. Once all the food and drinks have been served there should be some space for you to stand around and stretch near the food preparation area. If you explain to the airline staff that you have a back problem, they are normally very understanding.

Try to stretch your arms up high above your head. Circle and shrug your shoulders. Do some marching on the spot to keep your body from stiffening up.

Do not feel shy asking for assistance. Sometimes the aeroplane staff say they are not allowed to lift bags into the overhead lockers, so just ask a strong-looking passenger; most people are lovely and will be kind and help you. Most airlines offer an assistance service. Don't feel embarrassed to book this service; just enjoy the advantage that you skip the check-in queue and get whizzed through security.

AUTUMN

Fallen leaves are slippery. I never train clients outside on the pavements when they are covered in mulch. Take extra care and make sure your shoes grip. Certainly avoid running until the pavements are clear.

BAGS

Do not overload your bag. Some designer bags are really heavy even before you have added your contents.

Be mindful of how you carry a bag. Belt bags are really great as they put little stress on the shoulders and upper body. Rucksacks should be as light as possible. Use your pockets. Long periods of carrying on one side will most probably result in backache.

Gone are the days of dragging heavy school books around, but laptops can be heavy too. Ask for some help at school. The ideal solution would be to have one laptop/computer at school/work and another at home. Maybe ask friends to contribute to getting you a spare one.

BED

Recently a client asked for advice. She was in hospital for a separate procedure. She had to lie flat on her back and in her words 'It's killing me and nothing they're giving me helps.' (She is the client who suggested I include a Tips chapter in this guide.)

Sleeping on your back

Place a pillow under your thighs. It will take the pressure off your lower back. Also, a pillow between your legs and at either side of you for support so you can get cozy.

You may need two pillows under your thighs – just use trial and error to relieve the pressure.

In bed, as a relief, try hugging your knees in and circling your legs a little one way and then the other to try to massage your lower back.

Sleeping on your side

Put a cushion in between your thighs. This takes away the pressure of your upper leg collapsing onto your lower one causing the hips to go out of alignment and twisting and adding pressure to your lower spine. Place another cushion behind your back. Also one in front of your stomach, if that helps.

Sleeping on your front

This is not the best idea as your neck will be rotated to the side and often your back will arch. Just be mindful once you have had surgery.

There are many pillows and cushions available to buy. Just try some and see what works for you.

Getting out of bed

Avoid sitting straight up as this puts pressure on the lower spine.

Roll onto your side.

As you swing your legs over the side of the bed, walk your hands on the bed towards you to leverage yourself up until you are sitting upright on the side of the bed.

Mattress

The general advice from the stores is to get a soft mattress. A few years ago, it was generally recommended to purchase a hard one. Pre scoliosis surgery, make sure there is enough support for your curve without it being exaggerated by too soft a mattress. Post surgery, a soft mattress will mean that where the vertebrae are not fused there will be little support and too much pressure and instability. Go for a more supportive mattress, but not too solid. I am not big and prefer to sleep on a medium/hard mattress.

Some people like sleeping on a tempur mattress; hybrid mattresses are my personal choice.

BOWLING

Not really!

BRACE

If you have to wear a brace, try a really thin, good quality, extra-length vest with a high back so the plastic doesn't stick to you. Velvet, Splendid and Intimissi are brands that make comfortable vests. It is better to splash out on two or three of these as the comfort you will gain is worth the spend. Plus, if they are super-fine, they will dry quickly. In winter, use a baggy sweater or loose shirt that has length. In summer, A-line T-shirts or a pretty blouse will work best. If you want to wear a dress I would keep it boxy but short and wear it with strong gripping biker boots. Any stretchy leggings that sit low on your hips, so the band misses the start of your scar, will be good – jeans with a zip will be really uncomfortable.

For guys – same advice regarding vests. If you are keeping it casual, go for trackies and baggy tops. For suits, I would purchase a cheap one and go up a size, then bin it as soon as you get rid of your brace.

CLOTHES SHOPPING

I am also an experienced fashion stylist. Here are my 'scoliosis shopping tips'.

- Find a boutique you trust. You know where I am going with this one. You need someone who understands that a dress with a zipper down the back is going to look wonky on you. A romantic, full, pretty, off-the-shoulder top will make you look like you are about to take off! (I really hope that doesn't offend anyone.)

- Take your mum or your true best friend along – the one that says it like it is, not the one who says you look fantastic when you fear you look terrible.

- If you are brave enough, explain to the shop assistant you have an uneven back and that you really need an honest opinion. Tell the assistant you don't want to get home with your purchases and have to return them all because your family/friends tell you the clothes are not sitting in a flattering way. This will encourage the assistant to be truthful. (I have done this many times).

- If you are pre surgery your clothes choices are likely to be a bit more limited than post surgery.

One side will always be a little slimmer than the other. This is because your shoulder blade is likely to glide outwards over your ribs on one side, with the shoulder on that side of your curve slightly rotated forward. Anyone who does not have scoliosis may not understand this.

- Try to avoid tops and dresses with lots of seams that may draw attention to your lack of symmetry.

- Go for single-colour tops or small prints.

- Avoid very structured jackets if you are pre surgery – they won't sit right. Soft lines and fabrics that are fitted are more flattering.

- Crop tops look great over a fitted tank.

- Leggings or fitted trousers will draw attention to your legs and are more flattering.

- Avoid flowy tops with flowy trousers – too shapeless and unflattering.

- Asymmetrical clothing is a dream. A one-shoulder dress with the coverage on the side of the hump/uneven shoulder should look fabulous.

However hard it is to shop sometimes, please remember you may just be having a bad shopping day, which most people experience regularly – it's not just down to scoliosis. My friends with amazing bodies get depressed when everything looks awful on them and it is usually down to poorly cut clothes.

And always remember that that fabulous dress you saw online/on a celeb/model, etc., has been altered or pinned with bulldog clips at the back, as well as hair sprayed or glued to stay in place. That is why when you try it on in the shop's fitting room it looks nothing like the picture you saw – because it isn't! It has nothing to do with your scoliosis, pre or post surgery.

Clothes shopping for men

Before surgery my tips would include to avoid striped shirts and structured jackets with too many seams on the back. Try and stick to plain block colours. After surgery just wear comfortable trackies and baggy T-shirts/sweatshirts over your brace.

Once you have recovered and no longer need a brace just experiment with new shirt and jacket shapes to see what suits you and is comfortable.

SHOPPING FOR SHOES

I wear trainers most of the day. I do, however, love a high, elegant shoe. The main issue is the sole. Sadly, whatever the height or style, a cheap shoe will have a cheap sole with zero grip. If budget is an issue, purchase shoes in the sales or from a discount online store. In the winter, it is really important to have good, flat-heeled, sturdy boots that will grip the pavement. Biker-style boots usually tick that box. Guys, just look for shoes/trainers with a good grip.

DRIVING

Your rotation will be limited. When exiting a slip road onto a main road, take your time (you may need to shift your body to expand your visuals) and do not be rushed by other drivers. Wait until you feel safe to pull away.

EXERCISE/GYM CLASSES

There are some fantastic instructors out there who run incredible, fun classes. However, not all instructors will be aware of scoliosis and what is safe for you. Inform the instructor before the class and feel comfortable to just take part in some of the session. If in doubt, don't be afraid to sit the exercise out. Do a stretch instead. If an instructor is pushing you to do an exercise that does not feel right, please walk out. Keeping up with everyone else may result in an injury for you and lots of unnecessary pain and wasted time recovering.

In my opinion, I would avoid the following:

- Pumping any heavy weights in a class.
- Extreme aerobic moves.
- Jumping.
- Twisting.
- Boxercise in a class environment.
- Step classes – too much twisting.
- Any class where the instructor is just calling out the exercises and not checking on technique.

GOLF

This sport involves too much rotation. Avoid! I'm sorry. (See Tennis.)

GRABBER

This is an invaluable reaching tool which will reduce the need to bend or over-stretch. Use it for 'grabbing' things in high or hard-to-reach places.

HAIRDRESSING

My surgeon advised against this profession as it involves so much one-sided work and lots of hours standing with poor posture.

HOUSEWORK

The repetitive movement of one side of the body is a big no for scoliosis patients, before or after surgery. Before surgery, this is because you will build up the muscles on just one side of your body, depending on whether you are right- or left-handed. After surgery, because you can't! Your surgeon will most likely advise you not to clean/vacuum for up to six months after surgery. Try to get some cleaning help. Once you are fully recovered, and if you are not able to have any help with daily chores, keep changing your hands, especially when using a vacuum cleaner.

ICE SKATING

If you know how to skate, then it's up to you. Beginners, if you fall you will be very sore and could damage your back.

LAUNDRY

No, you are not crazy. T-shirts do get stretched out of shape with wear. Possibly yours do not look as symmetrical after being worn a few times as when you purchased them. Yes, this is partly due to scoliosis, but it is also down to the fact that most jersey fabric, unless it is super high quality, will twist after washing.

PARACHUTING

NEVER – no discussion, no advice, no alternatives.

PATTERN CUTTING

I had to stop this activity as I could no longer lean over a massive table to design a flat pattern. Draping a fabric to cut a pattern is a little less stressful but will still put pressure on the back. Mr Michael Edgar, my surgeon at the time, sadly advised me to change my career path.

PICKING UP STUFF

Always squat to pick up something from the floor, keeping your bottom higher than your knees. Hold your core in, use your glutes and quads, keeping your shoulders relaxed. Do not bend your knees lower than your bottom to crouch down as this movement will put pressure on your knees and if the object is heavy it is easy to use your back muscles and pull something out.

RISKY SPORTS AND EXPERIENCES

Why would you risk damaging yourself for a five-minute thrill? Check with your health insurance/holiday insurance policy if applicable to see if you would be covered. Yes, I know the majority of scoliosis patients are young and want to do fun sports with their friends, but take a breath (especially gap-year travellers) and decide if it's really worth it! White-water rafting, bungee jumping, mopeds, etc – I just don't see that any of this is worth the risk.

ROLLER COASTERS

NEVER – no alternatives.

Why? Apart from the stress on your spine and the possible damage from being shaken around, if you have had surgery you may not be insured. Most theme parks have a list of disclaimers and spinal surgery is usually included.

RUGBY

No, I'm afraid not – see the advice of orthopedic consultant Mr Michael Edgar (*Daily Mail*, 2002 www.dailymail.co.uk/health/article-102169/Whats-involved-spine-straightening.html/health/article-102169/Whats-involved-spine-straightening.html)

RUNNING

YES, BUT this is a tricky one. Most surgeons that I have come across (quite a few, if you count second and third opinions over the years) are not big fans. I am not massively keen. If you want to run, make sure you wear correct supportive trainers with moulded orthotic-style innersoles. Also make sure your trainers can bend – the cheaper ones and fashion trainers do not and this inhibits the flow of your feet when running, encouraging a flat-footed running style. You should not be able to hear your feet plonking down. If you can, there will be reverberations up to your spine.

Personally, and as a trainer, I would not encourage a client with scoliosis to run. My suggested time to wait is 18 months from the surgery date. Scoliosis patients, if you do choose to run, consult an experienced trainer who specialises in running/marathon training as the running style you adopt will make a huge difference to your back.

SHOPPING

Do your supermarket shopping online and/or use the shop's help-to-the-car services – or take a strong friend with you to the supermarket.

Try to carry your bags evenly – one on each side.

SHOWERS/HOT BATHS/WASHING HAIR

I always have a hot shower in the morning. I'm a huge believer in heat helping to soothe muscles. Many people prefer cold. It really is whatever works for you. I just find that, however stiff I feel, a shower helps.

When you have a bath – or are allowed a bath again a few months after surgery – be careful how you place your head to avoid straining your neck.

After surgery, your scar must not get wet. Ask the hospital to give you some massive waterproof dressings; they can also be ordered from your local pharmacy. I stood in the shower and my mum washed my hair. Once you are able to go a salon, tell the person washing your hair not to yank your head or to push the sink down hard onto your shoulders.

SHOW JUMPING

NEVER!

Horse riding is fine and at your own risk – just no jumps.

Orthopaedic consultant Mr Michael Edgar, my surgeon for the first two of my surgeries, was very clear on this point, together with parachuting and hairdressing.

SITTING

Try to sit symmetrically, with your hips balanced.

- Feet should be in front of knees.

- Do not tuck your feet under the chair – it puts too much pressure on your knees.

- Try putting a small cushion or a rolled-up scarf or sweatshirt under your glutes on the side where the hip sinks down. This will lift your body on that side and you will feel more comfortable and avoid lower backache.

- Do not be frightened of being fussy and asking to change your chair in a restaurant/at a friend's/at work. If the chair is too soft, the strain on your lower back where it is forced to arch may cause pain later.

- High-back wooden chairs tend to be uncomfortable.

- When you are reading/on social media/using a mobile phone or laptop, it is really best to avoid any position where your back is not supported correctly. Always try to work from a laptop sitting at a table. My pet hate is children or adults lying in bed, propped up by three pillows, with their thoracic spine (upper back) forcibly bent and head bent in a forward position. Five minutes like this will put strain on the vertebrae and neck. You or your child will probably be sore and also end up with a headache. Be very conscious of posture, especially when lying down. If you really want to work/read/watch something on a laptop in bed, then try always to sit with your lower back supported by pillows. Bend your knees and also put one or two pillows under them to take the pressure off your lower spine. Get up and walk around at least every 30 minutes.

SITTING STILL OR STANDING FOR LONG PERIODS

Avoid long periods of either; move around and stretch as much as you can.

SKIING

Yes, with caution; if you are an intermediate skier or above. Your twisting on turns will be limited.

You can wear a soft back support brace-belt for protection to cover your ribs. I have also tried the solid back protector braces. The ones I tried I found really uncomfortable – partly because they are mostly made for adult men or children, so none fitted me properly. Also, if you still have a hump it may sit weirdly. If you can get on with them, absolutely definitely use one.

Avoid holiday times when the slopes are crazy busy and you risk being knocked and bumped.

Avoid icy conditions and the black runs.

SUITCASES/TRAVELLING ALONE

Book 'Special assistance' at both ends of your train and plane journeys.

Even if you feel fully recovered post surgery, don't be shy to ask someone to help you take your case off the carousel in the Arrivals hall – better than attempting the move yourself and putting your back out.

SWIMMING

YES – Wonderful!

My surgeon had me swimming every day as soon as I took my brace off, six months after my first two surgeries. It tones your body. It is very safe – you really can't do much damage. Lovely for stretching too in the pool.

Just watch out with front crawl – I always find that, as my arms do not fully rotate, I end up swimming into other people! Ditto with backstroke.

TENNIS

Tennis is fine to play once fully recovered but check with your surgeon. Often the rotation of the shoulder on the concave side of the thoracic scoliosis is not smooth as the shoulder blade glides over the ribs. The shoulder is limited in its rotation, which will affect serving.

Remember to take into account that tennis is not a symmetrical sport and leans towards left- or right-sided muscle build up, depending on which hand is dominant.

This can cause an internal blister due to the uneven movement where the muscle rubs over the metal rods and screws which have been attached to the spine. It will not do any damage, just be a localised pain. I have personally experienced this. I stopped playing. If, however, tennis is your passion and the odd blister is worth it, then try to compensate by performing separate exercises using your lats (the two large back muscles with an insertion from the lower ribs to the shoulder) on the opposing side to your tennis arm.

The intense rotation of the body, reaching for balls, etc., in my opinion, puts needless stress on your body post surgery.

THEATRE/CINEMA

Use the child booster cushions often provided if the seats are old and too soft. Immediately post surgery, you may be too uncomfortable to sit for any length of time. Try waiting six months before you go. Don't worry about walking out if your back hurts. It's not worth suffering during and after.

WORKING FROM HOME

Move your shoulders and stretch your arms above your head every 15 minutes to keep pressure off your neck caused by looking down at your laptop and to help with posture. Set an alarm on your phone to remind you to get up every 45 minutes, walk around and do some stretches. Keep hydrated and go for at least one walk a day. Set aside 20 minutes to exercise in the morning or when your working day is over.

WORRYING/ANXIETY

Scoliosis can have a significant impact on mental health. Many of us are anxious and fearful. If this is true for you, please talk to your surgeon and GP to ask to be referred to a therapist rather than bottle it all up. The Scoliosis Association UK and groups outside the UK offer advice.

If you are suffering from any stress, anxiety or pain, Liz Bord recommends you try mindfulness meditation. John Kabat-Zinn (in *Full Catastrophe Living*, 1990) defined mindfulness as 'the awareness that arises from paying attention, on purpose, in the present moment and non-judgementally'. Liz says, 'In order to take control of your life, focus on your breath and sensations in your body; this will enable you to be in the present moment, not living in the past or worrying about the future. This helps with pain, both physical and emotional.'

CONCLUSION

I really hope that this guide helps you as someone with scoliosis, or as a physio or personal trainer, to understand what activities and exercises are okay for a scoliosis patient. Of course, this is all individual and I have to say again, please check with a qualified medical advisor before you perform any of these exercises or stretches.

Have fun picking out what works for you or your client, and which ones you like. I would love to hear from you so please contact me at:

info@scoliosishandbook.com
www.scoliosishandbook.com

Instagram
@scoliosishandbook

Facebook
Facebook.com/scoliosishandbook

Love,
Caroline X

Useful contacts

ASPIRE supporting people with spinal injury
020 8954 5759 • info@aspire.org.uk • aspire.org.uk

Aspire Leisure Centre
020 8954 5759 • reception@aspire.org.uk • www.aspireleisurecentre.org.uk

SAUK Scoliosis Association UK
helpline 020 8964 1166 • general enquiries 020 8964 5343
info@sauk.org.uk • sauk.org.uk

John Rutherford MCSP HCPC physiotherapist
020 7935 4750 / 07850699534
backpainspecialistslondon.co.uk

Liz Bord fitness instructor (cardiac rehab instructor)
07764946839 • fitnessgodess@hotmail.com

(All telephone numbers are +44 for the UK)

A note about the illustrations

Illustrations by the very talented Hannah
Robinson, who I can't thank enough for her
patience and attention to detail. Hannah says:

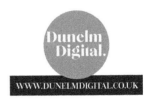

'I have always been passionate about marketing & graphic design, and love helping others achieve fantastic designs and illustrations that help their projects. It has been an absolute pleasure working with Caroline to bring her exercises to life in this book. She is a genuinely passionate and kind person. I can't wait to see how this book will help others.'

EXERCISE INDEX

For easy reference I have organised the exercises according to areas of the body being exercised. Most of the exercises overlap with different muscles but this index should help you find an exercise quickly. For example, under 'backs', a Lat pulldown exercise will also work your arms.

Please always check with your doctor/consultant/physiotherapist that these exercises are suitable for you.

GENERAL INDEX